Multiple Choice Questions for Operating Room and Critical Care Personnel

EMERGENCY CARE SERIES

Titles currently available:
Basic Concepts for Operating Room and Critical Care Personnel
S. J. Mather and D. L. Edbrooke

In Preparation:
Anaesthesia for Operating Room Personnel
S. J. Mather and D. L. Edbrooke

Clinical Handbook for Critical Care Personnel
S. J. Mather and D. L. Edbrooke

EMERGENCY CARE SERIES

Multiple Choice Questions for Operating Room and Critical Care Personnel

S. James Mather MB BS LRCP MRCS DRCOG FFARCS
Consultant Anaesthetist, Bassetlaw Health Authority
and
David L. Edbrooke LRCP MRCS FFARCS
Consultant Anaesthetist, Royal Hallamshire Hospital, Sheffield

WRIGHT · PSG
Bristol London Boston
1983

Published by
John Wright & Sons Ltd, 823–825 Bath Road, Bristol
BS4 5NU, England

John Wright PSG Inc.,
545 Great Road, Littleton, Massachusetts 01460, USA

British Library Cataloguing in Publication Data

Mather, S. J.
Multiple choice questions for operating room and critical care personnel.—(Emergency care series)
1. Operating room nursing 2. Intensive care nursing
I. Title II. Edbrooke, David L.
III. Series
610.73′677 RD32.3

ISBN 07236 0728 1

Library of Congress Catalog Card Number: 83–50628

Typeset and printed in Great Britain by
John Wright & Sons (Printing) Ltd, at The Stonebridge Press, Bristol

Preface

This book of multiple choice questions has been compiled to complement the 'Emergency Care Series' of textbooks published by John Wright & Sons. Every effort has been made to avoid ambiguity, a recurring problem in Q. & A. books. While opinion differs as to the treatment of many conditions, we have tried to reflect current trends is medical practice as far as possible. The responsibility for any error must be ours alone.

We would like to acknowledge the help given to us during the preparation of the manuscript by Lieut. J. E. Butter, RN REMT, Mr R. A. Warren FRCS, Mr J. R. Paskins FRCS, Dr G. Weston FFARCS and our secretaries Mrs B. Myers and Mrs A. Brady.

SJM
DLE

Contents

Questions

1. The type of bone tissue found on the outside of a bone is:

(a) Compact
(b) Cancellous
(c) Yellow bone marrow
(d) Red bone marrow

2. The medulla oblongata is part of the:

(a) Cerebrum
(b) Cerebellum
(c) Brain stem
(d) Spinal cord

3. The lining of the airways and fallopian tubes is:

(a) Squamous epithelium
(b) Transitional epithelium
(c) Ciliated epithelium
(d) Keratinized epithelium

4. The number of vertebrae in the spinal column is:

(a) 25
(b) 30
(c) 33
(d) 38

5. **Most of the energy for cellular activity is generated in the:**

(a) Endoplasmic reticulum
(b) Golgi apparatus
(c) Mitochondria
(d) Centrosomes

6. **Blood:**

(a) The white blood cells help to counteract infection
(b) A high level of potassium in the blood is likely to cause cardiac arrythmias
(c) Red blood cells contain iron
(d) Lymphocytes help to control blood clotting

7. **In cardiac physiology the following are true or false:**

(a) The sino-atrial node impulse initiates cardiac rhythm
(b) The performance of the left ventricle is partially determined by the left atrial filling pressure
(c) In atrial fibrillation the pulse is always regular
(d) Blood flows down the coronary arteries in diastole

8. **Cerebrospinal fluid is found between the:**

(a) Arachnoid mater and pia mater
(b) Pia mater and brain
(c) Dura mater and arachnoid mater
(d) Skull and dura mater

9. **In air the percentage of carbon dioxide is:**

(a) 4%
(b) 0·4%
(c) 0·04%
(d) 0·004%

10. **Which anaesthetic induction agent would be the most suitable to carry for major disasters:**

(a) Propanidid
(b) Thiopentone
(c) Althesin
(d) Ketamine

11. Rewarmed blood may be kept prior to use for:

(a) 3 minutes
(b) 30 minutes
(c) 3 hours
(d) 30 hours

12. Two 6-volt batteries joined in series will:

(a) Have a combined voltage of 6 volts
(b) Have a combined voltage of 12 volts
(c) Have the same voltage as two 6-volt batteries in parallel
(d) Have a variable voltage

13. Which of the following intravenous solutions could be described as a colloid:

(a) Blood
(b) Hartmann's solution
(c) Dextrose saline
(d) Dextran 70

14. Which of the following drugs would be of use in status asthmaticus:

(a) Propranolol
(b) Amphetamine
(c) Aminophylline
(d) Salbutamol

15. Cyanosis can be an indication of:

(a) Hypoxia
(b) Hypercarbia
(c) Poor perfusion
(d) Carbon monoxide poisoning

16. The colouring agent used with trichloroethylene is:

(a) Cremophor EL
(b) Waxolene blue
(c) Thymol
(d) Methylene blue

17. Which hormone controls the expulsion of milk from the female breast:

(a) Follicle stimulating hormone
(b) Luteinizing hormone
(c) Progesterone
(d) Oxytocin

18. What percentage of sodium is reabsorbed by the proximal convoluted tubule:

(a) 10%
(b) 20%
(c) 50%
(d) 80%

19. *β*-blocking drugs may:

(a) Be used in the treatment of angina pectoris
(b) Relieve the bronchospasm of asthma
(c) Be useful in the treatment of supraventricular dysrhythmias
(d) Be useful in patients with hypertension

20. Control of respiration involves:

(a) Osmoreceptors
(b) Baroreceptors
(c) Chemoreceptors
(d) The sino-atrial node

21. The functions of the kidney include:

(a) The production of urine
(b) The production of the hormone renin
(c) The production of antidiuretic hormone
(d) The production of the hormone erythropoietin

22. Which of the following statements about the rods and cones of the eye is true:

(a) Cones require higher light levels
(b) Rods are concerned with detailed and colour vision
(c) Rods perceive light generally and gross movement
(d) Rods require higher light levels

23. Which of the following bones occur in the ear:

(a) The hammer (malleus)
(b) The scaphoid
(c) The anvil (incus)
(d) The stirrup (stapes)

24. Which of the following bones is *not* in the skull:

(a) The temporal bone
(b) The ethmoid bone
(c) The frontal bone
(d) The sphenoid bone

25. The normal blood glucose level is:

(a) 5–10 mmol/l
(b) 15–20 mmol/l
(c) 25–30 mmol/l
(d) 35–40 mmol/l

26. What is the diastolic pressure in the left ventricle of the normal heart:

(a) 120 mmHg
(b) 80 mmHg
(c) 25 mmHg
(d) 0 mmHg

27. Which of the following statements are true about the measurement of pressure:

(a) Pressure is defined as force per unit area
(b) Pressure can be measured in kilopascals
(c) Pressure can be measured in Newtons per square metre
(d) Pressure can be defined as force per unit time

28. The percentage of oxygen in the air at 6000 m is:

(a) 26%
(b) 21%
(c) 16%
(d) 11%

29. The scaphoid bone is found in:

(a) The cervical spine
(b) The skull
(c) The wrist
(d) The ankle

30. In the arterial pressure wave the 'notch' on the downslope is called:

(a) The aortic notch
(b) The pulmonary notch
(c) The descending notch
(d) The dicrotic notch

31. A constituent of human blood which is a rich source of antibodies is:

(a) Thromboplastin
(b) Gamma-globulin
(c) Erythrocytes
(d) Thrombocytes (platelets)

32. A patient has blood belonging to group AB. He should be able to receive blood from:

(a) Group AB only
(b) Any blood group
(c) Groups A, B and AB only
(d) Groups AB and O only

32. The interior of the heart is lined with:

(a) Pericardium
(b) Endocardium
(c) Myometrium
(d) Endometrium

34. Which of the following arteries branch directly from the aorta:

(a) The radial arteries
(b) The vertebral arteries
(c) The coronary arteries
(d) The femoral arteries

35. Even if a person voluntarily holds his breath for as long as possible stimuli from the respiratory centre will reflexly make him breathe as a result of:

(a) Decreased blood oxygen level
(b) Increased blood oxygen level
(c) Increased blood carbon dioxide level
(d) Decreased blood carbon dioxide level

36. The following are effects of the sympathetic nervous system:

(a) Vasodilatation in the vessels of the gut
(b) Increasing force of contraction of the heart
(c) Constriction of the coronary arteries
(d) Bronchodilatation

37. The following are examples of proprioceptors:

(a) Muscle spindles
(b) Joint receptors
(c) Golgi tendon organs
(d) Baroreceptors

38. During swallowing, the opening into the trachea is normally reflexly covered by the:

(a) Glottis
(b) Epiglottis
(c) Larynx
(d) Pharynx

39. Computer memory can be stored on:

(a) Floppy disk
(b) A visual display unit (VDU)
(c) Magnetic tape
(d) Winchester disk

40. The knee joint is an example of a:

(a) Pivot joint
(b) Ball and socket joint
(c) Hinge joint
(d) Gliding joint

41. The nerve that controls and supplies the diaphragm is called:

(a) Glossopharyngeal nerve
(b) Phrenic nerve
(c) Digastric nerve
(d) Pharyngeal nerve

42. Blood is emptied into the heart from the inferior and superior venae cavae; this blood is:

(a) Deoxygenated and arterial
(b) Oxygenated and arterial
(c) Deoxygenated and venous
(d) Oxygenated and venous

43. Which of the following may be surrounded by a myelin sheath:

(a) Nerve cell body
(b) Axon
(c) Dendrites
(d) Neuroglia

44. The functions of the liver include:

(a) The production of bile
(b) The production of urea
(c) The production of plasma proteins
(d) The breakdown of many drugs

45. The chemical name for halothane is:

(a) 2-chloro-2-bromo-trifluoroethane
(b) 1-chloro-1-bromo-trifluoroethane
(c) 2-chloro-2-bromo-bifluoroethane
(d) 2-chloro-1-bromo-trifluoroethylene

46. Breakdown of which of the following releases the most energy in the body:

(a) 1 gram of carbohydrate
(b) 1 gram of vitamins
(c) 1 gram of fat
(d) 1 gram of protein

47. Which of the following statements is true:

(a) The right lung has three lobes
(b) The left lung has two lobes
(c) The circle of Willis is in the skull
(d) The islets of Langerhans are in the liver

48. In the electrocardiogram the 'P' wave corresponds to:

(a) Atrial contraction
(b) Atrial relaxation
(c) Conduction down the bundle of His
(d) Ventricular contraction

49. Spermatozoa are produced by:

(a) The testis
(b) The epididymis
(c) The seminal vesicles
(d) The prostate

50. The incubation period for hepatitis B is:

(a) 1 day
(b) 6 days
(c) 1 month
(d) 6 months

51. Which of the following non-depolarizing muscle relaxants was the first to be introduced into clinical practice:

(a) Alcuronium
(b) Pancuronium
(c) Gallamine
(d) *d*-Tubocurarine

52. Peristalsis in the gut is under the control of:

(a) The glossopharyngeal nerve
(b) Cranial nerve X
(c) Cranial nerve V
(d) The vagus nerve

53. Which hormone or hormones does the corpus luteum produce:

(a) Follicle stimulating hormone
(b) Luteinizing hormone
(c) Progesterone
(d) Oxytocin

54. A motor unit comprises:

(a) A motor neurone alone
(b) A motor and sensory neurone
(c) A sensory neurone and muscle fibre
(d) A motor neurone and muscle fibre

55. Which of the following organisms are Gram-positive:

(a) Staphylococci
(b) Proteus species
(c) Pertussis
(d) Tuberculosis

56. The autonomic nervous system issues from the spinal cord in outflows at the following levels:

(a) Cranial
(b) Cervical
(c) Thoracic
(d) Sacral

57. During massive transfusion, problems can arise with:

(a) Blood clotting
(b) Acidosis
(c) Hyperkalaemia
(d) Hypercalcaemia

58. In Britain the normal pressure in a full oxygen cylinder is approximately:

(a) 200 lbf/in^2
(b) 750 lbf/in^2
(c) 1000 lbf/in^2
(d) 2000 lbf/in^2

59. The pH of the gastric juice is normally:

(a) 1
(b) 4·7
(c) 7·4
(d) 11

60. Which of the following principles is used in the design of humidifiers:

(a) Vaporization
(b) Ultrasound
(c) Infra red radiation
(d) The Doppler effect

61. Which part of the brain controls posture and balance:

(a) The cortex
(b) The thalamus
(c) The hypothalamus
(d) The cerebellum

62. What is the systolic pressure in the right ventricle of the normal heart:

(a) 120 mmHg
(b) 80 mmHg
(c) 60 mmHg
(d) 25 mmHg

63. Which of the following drugs is *not* a diuretic:

(a) Frusemide
(b) Alcohol
(c) Chlorothiazide
(d) Chlormethiazole

64. The commonest blood group in the United Kingdom population is:

(a) Blood group A
(b) Blood group B
(c) Blood group AB
(d) Blood group O

65. The following drugs are useful in patients with pulmonary oedema:

(a) Frusemide
(b) Digoxin
(c) Hartmann's solution
(d) Oxygen

66. Acetylcholine is inactivated in a synapse by:

(a) GABA
(b) Serotonin
(c) Acetylcholinesterase
(d) Dopamine

67. Which of the following organisms are anaerobic:

(a) Staphylococci
(b) Tetanus bacilli
(c) Gas gangrene bacilli
(d) Tuberculosis bacilli

68. How many pairs of cranial nerves are there:

(a) 12
(b) 10
(c) 14
(d) 8

69. Which of the following drugs are bronchodilators:

(a) Aminophylline
(b) Atropine
(c) Isoprenaline
(d) Propranolol

70. The normal pH of the blood is approximately:

(a) 7·2
(b) 7·4
(c) 7·6
(d) 7·8

71. The strong fibrous membrane covering the bones is called:

(a) Cartilage
(b) Periosteum
(c) Articular surface
(d) Cancellous tissue

72. The brain stem and cerebellum:

(a) The cerebellum is responsible for control of posture and balance
(b) Lesions of the brain stem may result in an abnormal respiratory pattern
(c) A person with a cerebellar lesion may appear to be drunk
(d) The brain stem is necessary for life

73. How many orifices has the uterus:

(a) One
(b) Two
(c) Three
(d) Four

74. 1 gram of haemoglobin carries:

(a) 0·0139 ml oxygen
(b) 0·139 ml oxygen
(c) 1·39 ml oxygen
(d) 13·9 ml oxygen

75. Which of the following valves are situated on the right side of the heart:

(a) Aortic
(b) Tricuspid
(c) Mitral
(d) Pulmonary

76. The percentage of oxygen in expired air is:

(a) 14%
(b) 21%
(c) 16%
(d) 4%

77. During cell division the parts of the cell responsible for carrying over genetic material to the new cells are:

(a) Golgi apparatus
(b) Mitochondria
(c) Lysosomes
(d) Chromosomes

78. Which of the following are basic types of tissue:

(a) Connective
(b) Epithelial
(c) Gut
(d) Skin

79. The sino-atrial node is situated in the:

(a) Wall of the right atrium
(b) Interventricular septum
(c) Left atrium
(d) Wall of the right ventricle

80. Premature babies secrete:

(a) Too much surfactant
(b) Too little surfactant
(c) A normal amount of surfactant
(d) An abnormal type of surfactant

81. A resting adult requires:

(a) 25 ml of oxygen per minute
(b) 250 ml of oxygen per minute
(c) 2·5 litres of oxygen per minute
(d) 0·25 litres of oxygen per minute

82. The hip joint is an example of a:

(a) Pivot joint
(b) Ball and socket joint
(c) Hinge joint
(d) Gliding joint

83. Which of the following forces oppose the mean capillary pressure:

(a) Osmotic pressure of interstitial fluid
(b) Osmotic pressure of plasma proteins
(c) Interstitial fluid pressure
(d) Blood flow

84. The recurrent laryngeal nerve is a branch of the:

(a) Phrenic nerve
(b) The spinal accessory nerve
(c) The vagus nerve
(d) The hypoglossal nerve

85. The main types of lymphocytes include:

(a) B lymphocytes
(b) G lymphocytes
(c) T lymphocytes
(d) V lymphocytes

86. Which of the following pairs of words are synonymous:

(a) Anterior—ventral
(b) Posterior—ventral
(c) Superior—cranial
(d) Superior—caudal

87. The cell wall consists of a double layer of:

(a) Lipoprotein
(b) Deoxyribonucleic acid
(c) Ribonucleic acid
(d) Mitochondria

88. Haversian systems are found in the:

(a) Eye
(b) Bone
(c) Muscle
(d) Uterus

89. The functions of the skin include:

(a) Protection from excessive water loss
(b) Temperature regulation
(c) Perception of pain
(d) Protection from infection

90. Platelets are formed from:

(a) Lymphocytes
(b) Megakaryocytes
(c) A special type of red cell
(d) Mast cells

91. Which of the following bacteria are part of the clostridia group:

(a) *Viridans*
(b) *Welchii*
(c) *Pyocyaneus*
(d) *Tetani*

92. In what part of the body is the anvil found:

(a) The knee
(b) The ankle
(c) The eye
(d) The ear

93. Causes of hypokalaemia include:

(a) Malabsorption
(b) Diuretic therapy
(c) Blood transfusion
(d) Myocardial infarction

94. Which of the following is not an anticholinesterase:

(a) Pyridostigmine
(b) Scopolamine
(c) Neostigmine
(d) Edrophonium

95. The functions of the distal convoluted tubule include:

(a) Reabsorption of water
(b) Reabsorption of sodium ions
(c) Reabsorption of bicarbonate ions
(d) Reabsorption of food substances

96. Which of the following statements is correct:

(a) The pulmonary veins carry deoxygenated blood to the heart
(b) The pulmonary artery pressure is approximately 120/80 mmHg in a healthy adult
(c) In a person standing erect, the apex (top) of the lung has a greater blood supply than the base
(d) The mitral valve stands at the entrance to the aorta

97. Which cranial nerve controls movement of the pharynx:

(a) Cranial nerve II
(b) Cranial nerve IX
(c) The trigeminal
(d) The glossopharyngeal

98. The term used to denote a structure or position nearer to the centre line of the body is:

(a) Distal
(b) Superior
(c) Lateral
(d) Medial

99. Which of the following statements is true:

(a) The dura mater is outside the arachnoid mater
(b) The arachnoid mater is outside the pia mater
(c) The pia mater is inside the dura mater
(d) The arachnoid mater is inside the pia mater

100. If the heart muscle is stretched by extra blood filling it in diastole, it empties with more force on the next beat. This phenomenon is called:

(a) La Place's Law
(b) Starling's Law
(c) Poiseuille's Law
(d) Dalton's Law

101. The following number of vertebrae occur in the human spine:

(a) 7 cervical
(b) 7 thoracic
(c) 7 lumbar
(d) 7 coccygeal

102. In infants, total body water comprises the following percentage of body weight:

(a) 50%
(b) 60%
(c) 70%
(d) 80%

103. A normal blood pressure in a young person at rest might be:

(a) 99/55 mmHg
(b) 55/95 mmHg
(c) 10/6 cmHg
(d) 110/70 Torr

104. If all nerves to the heart were cut the heart would:

(a) Continue to beat
(b) Stop beating immediately
(c) Continue beating for a short period then stop
(d) Fibrillate

105. The foramen (hole) at the base of the skull through which the spinal cord enters is called:

(a) Foramen ovale
(b) Jugular foramen
(c) Occipital foramen
(d) Foramen magnum

106. A healthy adult at rest has a tidal volume of approximately:

(a) 500 ml
(b) 1000 ml
(c) 0·5 litres
(d) 5 litres

107. The function of the Nodes of Ranvier is to:

(a) Speed nerve conduction
(b) Slow nerve conduction
(c) Unknown
(d) Allow larger voltages to pass down the axons

108. Which of the following statements is true:

(a) Red blood cells carry oxygen
(b) White blood cells remain entirely within the vascular network
(c) Platelets are important in the clotting process
(d) White blood cells combat infections and clear debris from the body

109. Which of the following is *not* a chemical transmitter:

(a) Acetylcholine (ACh)
(b) Gamma aminobutyric acid (GABA)
(c) Acetylcholinesterase (AChE)
(d) 5-Hydroxytryptamine (Serotonin)

110. The vagus nerve's function is associated with:

(a) Smell
(b) Parasympathetic nerve supply to the heart and muscle of the gut
(c) Nerve supply to the vocal cords
(d) Movement of neck muscles

111. Which one of the following actions does the parasympathetic nervous system have:

(a) Inhibition of salivation
(b) Dilation of the pupil
(c) Accelerates the heart rate
(d) Constricts the bronchi

112. The kidneys receive the following percentage of the cardiac output:

(a) 0·2%
(b) 10%
(c) 25%
(d) 40%

113. Which of the following are involved in the maintenance of arterial blood pressure:

(a) The heart rate
(b) Good venous return
(c) Peripheral resistance
(d) Ventricular output

114. What happens when the diaphragm contracts:

(a) The diaphragm moves downwards enlarging the chest cavity
(b) Air is forced out of the lungs
(c) The diaphragm moves downward decreasing the size of the chest cavity
(d) Pressures within the chest increase

115. Which of the following lists the correct sequence of structures that air follows on inhalation:

(a) Larynx, trachea, pharynx, bronchi, epiglottis, alveoli
(b) Pharynx, larynx, epiglottis, alveoli, bronchi, trachea
(c) Pharynx, epiglottis, larynx, trachea, bronchi, alveoli
(d) Epiglottis, pharynx, larynx, trachea, bronchi, alveoli

116. Which of the following drugs are non-depolarizing muscle relaxants:

(a) Suxamethonium
(b) Alcuronium
(c) Decamethonium
(d) Pancuronium

117. Oxygen and carbon dioxide must be exchanged across the alveolar membrane in order to sustain life. This gas exchange occurs by:

(a) Diffusion
(b) Active transport
(c) Cellular pumps
(d) Effusion

118. Air sinuses are found in the following bones:

(a) Frontal
(b) Parietal
(c) Occipital
(d) Mastoid

119. Which of the following bones of the skull are moveable:

(a) Maxilla
(b) Mandible
(c) Malar
(d) Mastoid

120. Which of the following vitamins are water soluble:

(a) Vitamin A
(b) Vitamin B complex
(c) Vitamin C
(d) Vitamin D

121. The small intestine in man is approximately how long:

(a) 2·5 cm
(b) 2·5 m
(c) 25 m
(d) 250 m

122. Which of the following statements are theoretically true:

(a) A black body absorbs all the radiation falling on it
(b) A white body absorbs all the radiation falling on it
(c) A black body is a perfect radiator of heat
(d) A white body is a perfect radiator of heat

123. Which of the following hormones are produced in the anterior pituitary:

(a) Growth hormone
(b) Antidiuretic hormone
(c) Oxytocin
(d) Thyroid stimulating hormone

124. Cardiac arrest is characterized by:

(a) Pinpoint pupils
(b) Absent major pulses
(c) Warm dilated peripheries
(d) Cyanosis

125. Which of the following agents are intravenous anaesthetic induction agents:

(a) Thiopentone
(b) Ketamine
(c) Etomidate
(d) Althesin

126. Which of the following bones constitute a part of the pelvis:

(a) Ilium
(b) Ischium
(c) Pubis
(d) Sacrum

127. In an adult foreign bodies entering the trachea are most likely to end in:

(a) Left or right bronchus equally
(b) Neither left or right main bronchus
(c) Left main bronchus
(d) Right main bronchus

128. Which of the following drugs are diuretics:

(a) Propranolol
(b) Atracurium
(c) Mannitol
(d) Alcohol

129. Which of the following factors affect the glomerular filtration rate:

(a) Arterial blood pressure
(b) Venous blood pressure
(c) Osmotic effects of plasma proteins
(d) The pressure actually in Bowman's Capsule

130. Baroreceptor impulses tràvel along the:

(a) Vagus nerve
(b) Abducens nerve
(c) Glossopharyngeal nerve
(d) Spinal accessory nerve

131. Given that V is voltage, R is resistance, I is current, then Ohm's Law can be expressed as:

(a) $V = I.R$
(b) $V = I/R$
(c) $I = V/R$
(d) $VR = I$

132. Which of the following statements is true about erythropoietin:

(a) It is produced in the pancreas
(b) It is produced in the kidney
(c) It increases red blood cell formation
(d) It decreases red blood cell formation

133. Which of the following hormones are produced in the adrenal cortex:

(a) Mineralocorticoids
(b) Glucocorticoids
(c) Sex hormones
(d) Adrenaline

134. Which of the following are methods of measuring pressure:

(a) The Bourdon gauge
(b) The pneumotachograph
(c) Regnault's hygrometer
(d) The oscillotonometer

135. Which of the following drugs are sympathetic nervous system agonists:

(a) Adrenaline
(b) Dobutamine
(c) Isoprenaline
(d) Practolol

136. Hyaline cartilage:

(a) Is made up of elastic tissue
(b) Covers the ends of the bones in joints
(c) May become calcified
(d) Is harder than bone

137. The normal electrocardiogram:

(a) The P wave denotes atrial relaxation
(b) The QRS complex represents ventricular depolarization
(c) The T wave represents ventricular repolarization
(d) Contains an iso-electric line

138. Alternative current 'mains' electricity in the United Kingdom has the following characteristics:

(a) A frequency of 240 times per second
(b) A frequency of 50 times per second
(c) A voltage of 240 volts
(d) A voltage of 50 volts

139. The Venturi principle is used in the design of:

(a) Constant percentage oxygen master
(b) The bronchoscope injector
(c) The Bunsen burner
(d) Rotameters

140. The membranous space in the larynx where an emergency puncture can be made is called the:

(a) Crico-thyroid membrane
(b) Arytenoid membrane
(c) Thyrohyoid membrane
(d) Cricoid cartilage

141. Isotonic solutions have the same:

(a) Boiling points
(b) Osmotic pressures
(c) Surface tensions
(d) Solubility

142. The percentage of oxygen in air is approximately:

(a) 15%
(b) 21%
(c) 26%
(d) 31%

143. Which of the following anti-diabetic drugs are effective orally:

(a) Protamine zinc insulin
(b) Chlorpropramide
(c) Isophane insulin
(d) Tolbutamide

144. Which cranial nerve controls the pupil of the eye:

(a) I
(b) III
(c) V
(d) IX

145. Which one of these bones forms parts of the pelvic girdle:

(a) Clavicle
(b) Scapula
(c) Ilium
(d) Femur

146. Which of the following normal values are correct (for a 70 kg man):

(a) The vital capacity is approximately 4·5 litres
(b) The tidal volume is approximately 2·5 litres
(c) The functional residual capacity is approximately 0·5 litres
(d) The peak flow is approximately 3 litres/min

147. The normal number of parathyroid glands in the body is:

(a) 2
(b) 3
(c) 4
(d) 6

148. Which of the following drugs are specific H_2 receptor antagonists and thereby reduce gastric acidity:

(a) Magnesium trisilicate
(b) Carbenoxolone
(c) Cimetidine
(d) Ranitidine

149. The blood volume of a 70 kg man (11 stone) is approximately:

(a) 3 litres
(b) 5 litres
(c) 9 litres
(d) 11 litres

150. Which of the following drugs can be classified as benzodiazepines:

(a) Diazepam
(b) Chlordiazepoxide
(c) Nitrazepam
(d) Lorazepam

151. Control of respiration is from the respiratory centre which is located:

(a) In the cerebral cortex
(b) In the cerebellum
(c) In the vasomotor centre
(d) In the medulla oblongata

152. Which one of the following statements are correct:

(a) Cranial nerve I is the olfactory nerve and cranial nerve III is the optic
(b) Cranial nerve V is the trigeminal nerve and cranial nerve VII is the facial
(c) Cranial nerve XI is the vagus nerve and cranial nerve X is the glossopharyngeal
(d) Cranial nerve VI is facial and cranial nerve XII is the glossopharyngeal

153. Which of the following drugs are local analgesics:

(a) Bupivacaine
(b) Procaine
(c) Lignocaine
(d) Amethocaine

154. The vagus nerve is:

(a) Cranial nerve III
(b) Cranial nerve IX
(c) Cranial nerve XI
(d) Cranial nerve X

155. Which of the following statements are correct:

(a) Turbulent flow is faster than laminar flow
(b) Laminar flow has a parabolic wavefront
(c) Laminar flow speed is determined by the viscosity of the fluid
(d) Density determines the speed of turbulent flow

156. How many ribs articulate directly with the sternum:

(a) 7
(b) 10
(c) 14
(d) 20

157. Which of the following definitions are true:

(a) Pressure is force per unit area
(b) Energy is work per unit distance
(c) Momentum is mass per unit velocity
(d) Weight is the gravitational force acting on a body

158. The average stroke volume of the left ventricle is:

(a) 70 ml
(b) 70 ml/min
(c) 5 litres/min
(d) 5 litres

159. Which cranial nerves control eye movement:

(a) The optic nerve
(b) Cranial nerve III
(c) Cranial nerve VI
(d) The trochlear nerve

160. Which one of the following statements is correct:

(a) Transmission across a synapse is by electrical means
(b) Transmission across a synapse is by mechanical means
(c) Transmission across a synapse is by chemical means
(d) Transmission across a synapse is continuous

161. The first cervical vertebra is known as the:

(a) Scaphoid
(b) Ethmoid
(c) Axis
(d) Atlas

162. Which of the following are attributable to the actions of morphine:

(a) Euphoria
(b) Miosis
(c) Diarrhoea
(d) Depression of the cough reflex

163. A pH of 7·4 is equivalent to a hydrogen ion concentration of:

(a) 40 hydrogen ions per litre
(b) 4×10^6 hydrogen ions per litre
(c) 40×10^9 hydrogen ions per litre
(d) 40×10^6 hydrogen ions per litre

164. Which of the following are attributable to the actions of aspirin:

(a) Lowering of body temperature
(b) Respiratory depression
(c) Increased bleeding tendency
(d) Mucosal damage in the gastrointestinal tract

165. Which of the following principles have been used in devices for measuring flow:

(a) Ultrasound
(b) Faraday's Law
(c) Dalton's Law of partial pressures
(d) Thermodilution

166. Which of the following drugs are commonly referred to as 'controlled drugs' (under the Misuse of Drugs Act)

(a) Diamorphine
(b) Dihydrocodeine injection
(c) Pentazocine
(d) Pethidine

167. Which of the following effects are mediated by the parasympathetic nervous system:

(a) Decrease in the heart rate
(b) Dilatation of the bronchi
(c) Salivation
(d) Constriction of the pupils of the eye

168. A mole is:

(a) The atomic weight of a substance in milligrams
(b) The molecular weight of a substance in milligrams
(c) The atomic weight of a substance in grams
(d) The molecular weight of a substance in grams

169. Which of the following drugs are steroids:

(a) Cortisone
(b) Methylprednisolone
(c) Chlorpropramide
(d) Fludrocortisone

170. Which of the following antibiotics can cause damage to cranial nerve VIII:

(a) Penicillin
(b) Cephaloridine
(c) Gentamicin
(d) Nystatin

171. Tuberculosis can be spread by:

(a) Droplet infection
(b) Direct contact
(c) Mosquitoes
(d) Infected milk

172. It is theoretically possible to liquefy which of the following gases:

(a) Oxygen
(b) Nitrous oxide
(c) Nitrogen
(d) Carbon dioxide

173. The functions of the proximal convoluted tubule of the kidney include:

(a) Reabsorption of sodium ions
(b) Passive secretion of hydrogen ions
(c) Reabsorption of bicarbonate
(d) Reabsorption of food substances

174. Which of the following are units of work:

(a) Joule
(b) Newton-metre
(c) Pascal
(d) Joules per second

175. Which of the following drugs characteristically cause an increase in heart rate:

(a) Isoprenaline
(b) Pancuronium
(c) Methylprednisolone
(d) Atropine

176. Which of the following drugs are parasympathetic antagonists:

(a) Atropine
(b) Neostigmine
(c) Dobutamine
(d) Glycopyrollate

177. Which of the following act as buffering ions in a buffer system:

(a) Bicarbonate
(b) Phosphate
(c) Protein
(d) Hydrogen ions

178. Which of the following statements are true:

(a) Oxygen tension is expressed as a percentage
(b) Oxygen saturation is expressed in kilopascals
(c) Oxygen content is expressed in ml of oxygen per 100 ml of blood
(d) Oxygen saturation is expressed as a percentage

179. Which of the following statements about flow is true:

(a) Flow can be expressed in cubic metres per second
(b) Turbulent flow is dependent upon the viscosity of the fluid rather than density
(c) Laminar flow is dependent upon the viscosity of the fluid rather than density
(d) Flow can be measured using a pneumotachograph

180. Which of the following are computer programming languages:

(a) Pascal
(b) Byte
(c) Fortran
(d) Cobol

181. Which of the following products are produced from blood:

(a) Platelet concentrate
(b) Albumen
(c) Plasma protein fraction
(d) Dextran

182. Which of the following drugs are oral antidiabetic drugs:

(a) Chlorpropramide
(b) Phenformin
(c) Isophane insulin
(d) Primidone

183. Which of the following effects would occur by stimulation of the adrenal medulla:

(a) Constriction of the pupils of the eye
(b) Constriction of muscle blood vessels
(c) Dilatation of bronchioles
(d) Reduction of peristalsis

184. The parameters on the axes of the oxyhaemoglobin dissociation curve are:

(a) Oxygen content and oxygen tension
(b) Saturation of haemoglobin and oxygen tension
(c) Saturation of haemoglobin and oxygen content
(d) Carbon dioxide tension and saturation of haemoglobin

185. Which of the following drugs are narcotic antagonists:

(a) Naloxone
(b) Nefopam
(c) Nalorphine
(d) Nikethamide

186. Humidity can be measured using:

(a) Regnault's hygrometer
(b) A thermocouple
(c) The hair hygrometer
(d) The wet and dry bulb hygrometer

187. The peak flow in a 70 kg man is approximately:

(a) 600 ml per minute
(b) 6 litres per minute
(c) 60 litres per minute
(d) 600 litres per minute

188. Which of the following drugs affects the synthesis of noradrenaline:

(a) Guanethidine
(b) Labetolol
(c) α-methyldopa
(d) Trimetaphan

189. Waste products excreted in the urine are:

(a) Urea
(b) Uric acid
(c) Cholesterol
(d) Creatinine

190. In the brain the cerebellum controls:

(a) Memory and speech
(b) Posture and balance
(c) Voluntary movement in the lower half of the body
(d) Involuntary sphincters

191. The bones which make up the toes are called:

(a) Metacarpals
(b) Metatarsals
(c) Tarsals
(d) Phalanges

192. Which of the following statements are true:

(a) There are normally four pineal glands
(b) A Graafian follicle is found in the testis
(c) The uvula is part of the kidney
(d) The middle ear controls balance and posture

193. Organs which are important in the elimination of an acid load include:

(a) The brain
(b) The pancreas
(c) The kidney
(d) The lung

194. Which of the following drugs are hypnotics:

(a) Chlordiazepoxide
(b) Glycopyrrolate
(c) Nitrazepam
(d) Mannitol

195. Which of the following normal values are approximately correct (for a 70 kg man):

(a) The stroke volume is 70 ml
(b) The plasma sodium is 140 mmol/l
(c) The haemoglobin is 14 g/100 ml of blood
(d) The partial pressure of oxygen in arterial blood is 5 kPa

196. Which of the following drugs are used to treat hypertension:

(a) Cimetidene
(b) Propranolol
(c) Noradrenaline
(d) Methyldopa

197. Which of the following are properties of pure trichloroethylene:

(a) It has a blue colour
(b) It is a good analgesic
(c) It is best used in closed circuit anaesthesia
(d) Recovery from anaesthesia with this agent is slow

198. Which vitamin is necessary for blood clotting:

(a) Vitamin A
(b) Vitamin D
(c) Vitamin E
(d) Vitamin K

199. Which of the following values, expressed as a percentage of body weight (in an adult), are correct:

(a) Intracellular fluid 45%
(b) Interstitial fluid 13%
(c) Plasma 20%
(d) Extracellular fluid 17%

200. Which of the following statements are true:

(a) 212 °F is equivalent to 100 °C
(b) The boiling point of water at sea level is 98·4 °F
(c) Freezing of water occurs at 38 °F
(d) The normal body temperature is 37 °C

201. Stones (calculi) in the bile duct may cause:

(a) Generalized abdominal pain
(b) Pain in the shoulder tip
(c) Epistaxis
(d) Jaundice

202. Infected urine may result in:

(a) Haematuria (blood in the urine)
(b) Pain on passing urine
(c) Loin pain
(d) Shoulder tip pain

203. Aortic aneurysm may:

(a) Lead to sudden death
(b) Give rise to severe back pain
(c) Cause renal failure
(d) Lead to ulnar nerve palsy

204. Cardiac pacemakers which are nuclear-powered:

(a) May be a radiation hazard to the wearer
(b) May not be left in the body following death and cremation.
(c) Have a shorter life but are less bulky than those with conventional batteries
(d) Can only be worn externally

205. An obstructed airway is suggested by:

(a) Indrawing of tissue between the ribs (intercostal recession)
(b) Rhythmic movements of the abdominal wall without obvious indrawing of breath
(c) Slow, deep respiration
(d) Stridor

206. Tumours of the lung and pleura are associated with:

(a) Smoking tobacco
(b) Smoking cannabis
(c) Asbestosis
(d) Emphysema

207. Respiratory failure is characterized by:

(a) Drowsiness
(b) Decreased arterial oxygen tension
(c) Vomiting
(d) Convulsions

208. In the first 6 hours following myocardial infarction the ECG often shows:

(a) Elevated S–T segments
(b) Flattened T waves
(c) Inverted P waves
(d) Tall, peaked T waves

209. In left ventricular failure the patient is short of breath due to:

(a) Pulmonary oedema
(b) Pulmonary infarction (death of lung tissue)
(c) Poor coronary blood flow
(d) Inadequate venous return to the right heart

210. Sudden cessation of steroid therapy in a patient who has taken these drugs for a long time may:

(a) Result in acute renal failure
(b) Result in an 'adrenal (Addisonian) crisis'
(c) Lead to hypotension (low blood pressure)
(d) Lead to hypertension (high blood pressure)

211. Coumarin anti-coagulant drugs:

(a) Work by preventing synthesis of vitamin E
(b) Can be antagonized by vitamin K
(c) In overdosage may lead to cerebral haemorrhage
(d) Are only active by injection

212. Chronic bronchitis in adults is associated with:

(a) Smoking
(b) Living at altitude
(c) Emphysema
(d) Urban pollution

213. Which of the following are true:

(a) An oropharyngeal airway may be inserted in a conscious patient
(b) Intubation should always be attempted in cases of respiratory arrest
(c) Defibrillation is more likely to succeed in the case of 'coarse' rather than 'fine' ventricular fibrillation
(d) Sinus arrhythmia is potentially life-threatening if untreated

214. Which of the following statements are correct:

(a) Intubation should always be preceded by ventilation with oxygen
(b) Absent breath sounds following intubation may be ignored if the chest wall moves with ventilation
(c) Emergency tracheostomy should be carried out at the level of the cricoid cartilage
(d) Inhaled foreign bodies tend to enter the right lung in adult

215. Endotracheal suction may:

(a) Cause cardiac dysrhythmia
(b) Cause bronchospasm
(c) Cause laryngospasm
(d) Cause arterial hypoxia

216. In drowning:

(a) Mechanical methods of artificial ventilation (Holger-Nielsen) are better than mouth-to-mouth methods because of the water in the lungs
(b) Whilst the patient is still in the water it is essential to perform cardiac massage before artificial ventilation
(c) A fall into very cold water can produce death from cardiac arrest without water entering the lungs
(d) Pink froth at the patient's mouth shows that death occurred more than an hour before

217. Decompression sickness or 'the bends':

(a) Can only be treated in a decompression chamber
(b) Can be treated with high dose steroids alone
(c) Is due to oxygen coming out of solution in the tissue
(d) Can also occur at high altitude

218. A patient who is suffering from exposure will:

(a) Have a higher than normal body temperature
(b) Always be deeply cyanosed
(c) Probably have visual disturbances
(d) Probably have slurred speech

219. Treatment for exposure should include:

(a) Alcohol by mouth
(b) Exposure of the head and neck region
(c) Putting the patient's feet above level of heart
(d) Re-warming

220. Early treatment for frostbite should be by:

(a) Re-warming in a hot bath (over 40 °C)
(b) Vigorous rubbing or beating of the affected part
(c) Local application of alcohol
(d) Application of snow or ice to proximal parts of the affected limb

221. The heart rate may be increased by which of the following drugs:

(a) Propranolol
(b) Adrenaline
(c) Glycopyrrolate
(d) Insulin

222. Bronchospasm may be relieved by:

(a) Atropine
(b) Isoprenaline
(c) Salbutamol
(d) Hydrocortisone

223. Sodium bicarbonate may:

(a) Be used to treat metabolic acidosis
(b) Worsen congestive cardiac failure
(c) Raise serum potassium levels
(d) Cause a transient rise in $Paco_2$

224. Nitrous oxide (as Entonox) should not be administered to:

(a) Children
(b) Patients with a suspected pneumothorax
(c) Patients with head injuries
(d) Patients with myocardial infarction

225. The following solutions are isotonic with plasma:

(a) Ringer-lactate (Hartmann's solution)
(b) Dextran 110 in 5% dextrose
(c) Haemaccel (gelatin solution)
(d) 10% Dextrose solution

226. In haemorrhagic shock, symptoms and signs are due to:

(a) Hypothermia
(b) Hypovolaemia
(c) Hypotension
(d) Hyperpnoea

227. Which of the following conditions constitute an increased anaesthetic risk:

(a) Kyphoscoliosis
(b) Sickle cell anaemia
(c) Hypertension
(d) Patients regularly taking night sedation

228. Intravenous infusion of a plasma 'volume expander' such as Dextran 70 is indicated in:

(a) Congestive cardiac failure
(b) Hypovolaemia
(c) Pulmonary oedema
(d) Chronic renal failure

229. Traumatic injury to the abdomen may result in:

(a) Internal haemorrhage
(b) Ruptured stomach
(c) Pain at the shoulder tip
(d) Blood in the urine

230. The following drugs are useful in the treatment of most cases of anaphylactic shock:

(a) Adrenaline
(b) Practolol
(c) Digoxin
(d) Hydrocortisone

231. Modern treatment of acute epiglottitis in children may include:

(a) Humidification of inspired gases
(b) Awake intubation
(c) Antibiotics
(d) General anaesthesia

232. Treatment of drowned casualties may include:

(a) Cardiac massage
(b) Endotracheal intubation
(c) Intravenous sodium bicarbonate
(d) Intravenous steroid therapy

233. The objectives of the preoperative visit by the anaesthetist are:

(a) To assess the need for and prescribe premedication
(b) To assess the patient's physical status
(c) To explain the anaesthetic procedure to the patient
(d) To reduce the risk of mistaken identity

234. Decompression sickness may be manifest as:

(a) Pain, flitting from joint to joint
(b) Unexplained malaise and nausea
(c) Vertigo and difficulty in speaking
(d) Breathlessness, accompanied by chest pain

235. The treatment of status asthmaticus may include:

(a) Oxygen given by mask
(b) Intravenous bronchodilators
(c) Intravenous steroid therapy
(d) Intermittent positive pressure ventilation

236. Drug overdose commonly results in:

(a) Depressed conscious level
(b) Respiratory depression
(c) Increased production of urine
(d) Hypothermia

237. In drowning, death may occur due to:

(a) Hyperkalaemia (high plasma potassium)
(b) Pulmonary oedema
(c) Hypoxia
(d) Sodium overload (hypernatraemia)

238. Nitrous oxide (as Entonox) is a safe analgesic in the following conditions:

(a) Myocardial infarction
(b) Decompression sickness (the bends)
(c) Fractured ribs with pneumothorax
(d) Renal colic

239. Which of the following statements regarding ventricular fibrillation are true:

(a) It is associated with a cardiac output of about 2 litres per minute
(b) It is possible to feel the fibrillation by putting a hand on the chest
(c) It may be reverted to sinus rhythm by defibrillation
(d) It can be successfully treated by 100% oxygen

240. A Colle's fracture involves which of the following bones:

(a) Radius
(b) Femur
(c) Tibia
(d) Humerus

241. A Smith's fracture involves which of the following:

(a) Femur
(b) Fibula
(c) Ulna
(d) Radius

242. A Pott's fracture involves which of the following bones:

(a) Humerus
(b) Radius
(c) Tibia
(d) Ulna

243. Which of the following veins is it feasible to cannulate percutaneously:

(a) The basilic
(b) The internal jugular
(c) The femoral
(d) The azygos

244. Which of the following statements about high velocity bullet injuries are true:

(a) As the speed of entry is much greater, and the bullet tends to pass through the tissue, less tissue damage will occur
(b) The tissue involved is often viable
(c) The injuries involved are more easily dealt with than low velocity bullet injuries
(d) Widespread tissue damage may occur remote from the bullet track

245. A child has drunk a small quantity of turpentine from a carelessly placed bottle:

(a) The child should be made to vomit immediately by sticking a finger into the throat
(b) A drink of warm salty water should be given
(c) A drink of milk should be given
(d) His clothes should be removed and the skin around the face and chest washed

246. A young child has spilt scalding water all over himself:

(a) His clothes should be removed immediately and he should be placed in a bath of cold water
(b) He should immediately be placed in a bath of cold water before waiting to remove his clothes
(c) The child should be wrapped in a warm blanket before transfer to hospital
(d) A scald from boiling water is usually more dangerous and penetrating than a 'dry' burn, e.g. from falling against a bonfire

247. An old lady slips and falls on her hand. Her wrist is swollen, painful and looks deformed:

(a) Her arm should be put in a broad-arm sling
(b) Her arm should be held in a collar-and-cuff
(c) A nice hot cup of tea would be a good idea for the old lady
(d) She should be asked if she takes any tablets or medicines and to take them to the hospital with her

248. A child is choking after inhaling a marble. He is coughing and spluttering and in discomfort but is conscious and managing to breathe—one should:

(a) Encourage the child to drink a glass of milk
(b) Put one's fingers into his throat to try to get out the marble
(c) Do nothing other than rush him to hospital immediately
(d) Perform the Heimlich manoeuvre

249. Following an accident, there is a large wound to the foot which is bleeding profusely:

(a) A tourniquet should be applied tightly above the wound and left there
(b) A tourniquet should be applied moderately tightly and released every 10 minutes
(c) A pad should be pressed firmly over the bleeding wound
(d) No unsterile material must be allowed near the wound for fear of infection

250. A subarachnoid local anaesthetic block is produced by injecting the drug:

(a) Into a vein
(b) Into the cerebrospinal fluid
(c) Into the epidural space
(d) Under the sacrococcygeal ligament

251. Which of the following diseases can cause problems for the anaesthetist:

(a) Ankylosing spondylitis
(b) Malignant hyperpyrexia
(c) Hypertension
(d) Diabetes mellitus

252. Following inhalation of vomit, the first action the anaesthetist should take is:

(a) To give large doses of steroids intravenously
(b) Start a course of antibiotics
(c) Try to suck out the vomit through a bronchoscope
(d) Intubate the patient

253. The pH of freshly drawn human blood is normally around:

(a) 6·4
(b) 7·4
(c) 7·8
(d) 8·4

254. Which of the following is not a laryngoscope:

(a) Magill
(b) Mackintosh
(c) Robert Shaw
(d) Foley

255. Which of the following induction agents is least suitable for day case surgery:

(a) Methohexitone
(b) Thiopentone
(c) Etomidate
(d) Althesin

256. The pressure generated in the circuit when ventilating a patient with normal lungs is typically:

(a) 20 lbf/in^2
(b) 20 cmH_2O
(c) 20 mmHg
(d) 20 kPa

257. During laparoscopy, which of the following complications may occur:

(a) CO_2 embolism
(b) Hypotension
(c) Acute retention of urine
(d) Phrenic nerve palsy

258. The following drugs are used to induce hypotension for surgery:

(a) Halothane
(b) Sodium nitroprusside
(c) Nitroglycerine
(d) Promethazine

259. The following are recognized complications of hypotensive techniques:

(a) Cerebrovascular accident (stroke)
(b) Delayed recovery from anaesthesia
(c) Renal failure
(d) Impairment of liver function for several days

260. In hyperkalaemia (high plasma potassium concentration), the ECG may have the following changes:

(a) Flattened P wave
(b) Flattened T wave
(c) Tall peaked P wave
(d) Tall peaked T wave

261. In a child weighing 10 kg the most suitable circuit for inhalation anaesthesia with spontaneous respiration would be:

(a) Bain (Mapleson D)
(b) Magill (Mapleson A)
(c) T-piece (Mapleson E)
(d) Lack (Mapleson A)

262. Epidural analgesia is suitable for:

(a) Intra-operative and postoperative pain relief in cholecystectomy
(b) Trans-urethral resection of the prostate gland
(c) Thyroidectomy
(d) Analgesia in a patient with fractured ribs

263. The following are contra-indications to the placement of an epidural cannula:

(a) Pre-existing neurological disorder
(b) Anticoagulant therapy
(c) Local sepsis
(d) Concurrent treatment with opiate analgesics

264. Axillary brachial plexus block may be complicated by:

(a) Haematoma
(b) Pneumothorax
(c) Peripheral nerve injury
(d) Horner's syndrome (due to sympathetic ganglion block)

265. It is important to remove make-up and nail varnish preoperatively because:

(a) It can cause cross infection by adhering to the anaesthetic apparatus
(b) May obscure physical signs
(c) May react chemically with the anaesthetic agents
(d) Can cause skin irritation following anaesthesia

266. The pH of citrated (bank) blood is around:

(a) 5·8
(b) 6·8
(c) 7·8
(d) 8·8

267. During thyroidectomy there is a risk of damage to:

(a) The facial nerve
(b) The phrenic nerve
(c) The recurrent laryngeal nerve
(d) The brachial plexus

268. The pregnant patient at term has:

(a) An increased blood volume
(b) An increased haemoglobin concentration
(c) Increased oxygen consumption
(d) Increased $Paco_2$

269. Apgar scoring is used in the assessment of:

(a) Coma
(b) Chronic bronchitis
(c) The newborn
(d) Diabetes

270. Which of the following drugs are used for premedication:

(a) Lorazepam
(b) Pancuronium
(c) Atropine
(d) Papaveretum

271. The central venous pressure is equivalent to pressure in:

(a) The left atrium
(b) The right atrium
(c) The left ventricle
(d) The right ventricle

272. Which of the following are signs of severe dehydration:

(a) Decreased skin elasticity
(b) Hypotension
(c) Poor peripheral perfusion
(d) Low urine output

273. In general anaesthesia for day case surgery, it is:

(a) Mandatory for the patient to be accompanied home
(b) Permissible for the patient to drive himself home
(c) Not necessary for the patient to be assessed by the anaesthetist before the anaesthetic
(d) Permissible for the patient to drink up to 500 ml of liquid 2 hours before operation provided he has not eaten

274. In those exposed to waste anaesthetic gases over a long period there is said to be:

(a) An increased incidence of spontaneous abortion
(b) An increased incidence of congenital malformation of fetuses
(c) A tendency to diabetes
(d) An increased incidence of sterility in males

275. During anaesthesia for thoracic surgery, cardiac arrhythmias may occur due to:

(a) Traction on the vagus nerves
(b) Compression of the heart and great vessels
(c) Compression of the adrenal gland
(d) Spreading of ribs to gain access to the thorax

276. In patients with mitral stenosis induction of anaesthesia should be slow because:

(a) The cardiac output is relatively fixed
(b) Myocardial depression may be severe
(c) Most of the cardiac output is directed to the brain
(d) Ventricular fibrillation may follow

277. Ethylene oxide sterilization:

(a) Is safe for anaesthetic equipment that would be damaged by intense heat and moisture
(b) Kills tubercule bacillus
(c) Readily penetrates rubber and plastic
(d) Kills all pathogenic bacteria at room temperature

278. Signs associated with cardiac tamponade are:

(a) Low blood pressure
(b) Distended neck veins
(c) Distant or inaudible heart sounds
(d) Profound respiratory difficulty

279. 'Flail chest' is associated with:

(a) Blunt trauma to the thorax
(b) Paradoxical respiration
(c) Hypoxia
(d) Haematuria

280. Immediate care of a flail chest includes:

(a) Splinting the flail segment
(b) Lying the patient on the affected side
(c) Lying the patient on the opposite side
(d) Administration of 1 litre of whole blood as soon as possible

281. Shock lung (adult respiratory distress syndrome) may follow:

(a) Blast injury
(b) Burns
(c) Massive blood transfusion
(d) Blunt chest trauma

282. Reliable routes for administration of drugs at the accident site are:

(a) By inhalation
(b) By intravenous injection
(c) By intramuscular injection
(d) Rectally

283. The most common type of head injury is that caused by:

(a) Acceleration/deceleration
(b) Crushing injury
(c) Penetrating wound
(d) Direct violence

284. The ideal position in which to transport a *conscious* patient with a suspected cervical spine fracture is:

(a) Sitting, head flexed
(b) Sitting, head extended
(c) Prone, with one pillow
(d) Supine, neck splinted in neutral position

285. Features of tension pneumothorax include:

(a) Increasing breathlessness
(b) Small volume pulse
(c) Loss of breath sounds over the affected side
(d) Displacement of the apex beat toward the affected side

286. Sweating is a characteristic of:

(a) Belladonna poisoning
(b) Anxiety states
(c) Hypovolaemic shock
(d) Severe pain

287. Cardiac output usually increases in:

(a) Thyrotoxicosis
(b) Myocardial infarction
(c) Exercise
(d) 'Addisonian crisis' (lack of steroid hormones in adrenal failure)

288. Rheumatic fever:

(a) May affect the heart valves
(b) May affect the kidney
(c) Follows infection with certain strains of streptococci
(d) May affect the nervous system producing abnormal movement (chorea)

289. D.C. shock is useful in the following conditions:

(a) Asystole
(b) Ventricular fibrillation
(c) Atrial fibrillation
(d) Heart block

290. Bronchospasm (wheezing) may often be precipitated in asthmatics by:

(a) Exposure to house dust
(b) Infection
(c) Alcohol
(d) Emotional disturbances

291. Tuberculosis:

(a) Can only be contracted from cow's milk which is unpasteurized
(b) Is caused by a virus
(c) Can be treated with antibiotics
(d) Is always confined to the lungs

292. Emphysema results in:

(a) Obstructive airways disease
(b) An increase in P_{CO_2} in most cases
(c) Peripheral cyanosis
(d) Chronic bronchitis

293. Spontaneous pneumothorax:

(a) Characteristically occurs in the elderly
(b) Usually produces 'pleuritic' type chest pain (worse on inspiration)
(c) Suggests underlying severe lung disease
(d) Often recurs

294. The following are characteristics of aspirin overdose:

(a) Tinnitus (ringing in the ears)
(b) Unconsciousness
(c) Rapid respiration
(d) Clammy skin

295. The following *regularly* occur in paracetamol poisoning:

(a) Very early liver failure with jaundice
(b) Renal failure
(c) Coma
(d) Profuse diarrhoea

296. Bronchiectasis means:

(a) Dilatation of the bronchi due to disease
(b) Dilatation of the bronchial veins
(c) Constriction of the alveolar ducts
(d) Collapse of the alveoli

297. In a young asthmatic, the following would be characteristic of an asthmatic attack:

(a) Retention of carbon dioxide (raised P_{CO_2})
(b) Moderate hypoxia
(c) Immediate improvement when steroids are administered intravenously
(d) Good response to bronchodilators

298. Paraquat poisoning results in:

(a) Gastrointestinal irritation and bleeding
(b) Liver damage
(c) Renal damage
(d) Inflammation of the alveoli

299. Toadstool poisoning by the Death Cap Fungus (*Amanita* sp.) results in:

(a) Abdominal pain and bleeding per rectum
(b) Diarrhoea
(c) Cardiac failure
(d) Tetany

300. Which of the following drugs are usually used to treat ventricular extrasystoles:

(a) Practolol
(b) Atropine
(c) Lignocaine
(d) Disopyramide

301. A pneumothorax can be caused by:

(a) Coughing
(b) Artificial ventilation of the lungs
(c) Severe hypoxia
(d) Epileptic fits

302. Severe and prolonged vomiting can lead to:

(a) Alkalosis
(b) Acidosis
(c) Dehydration
(d) Heart failure

303. Indications of severe abdominal trauma may include:

(a) Increasing girth
(b) A painful rigid abdomen
(c) A falling haemoglobin
(d) Blurred vision

304. One pint (560 ml) of blood will cover an area approximately:

(a) 1 square foot
(b) 4 square feet
(c) 8 square feet
(d) 12 square feet

305. The effects of iron poisoning include:

(a) Vomiting
(b) Diarrhoea
(c) Convulsions
(d) Abnormally high haemoglobin level

306. Trauma victims may suffer acute respiratory embarrassment due to:

(a) Acute gastric dilatation
(b) Diaphragmatic rupture
(c) Fractured spine
(d) Femoral hernia

307. Which of the following increase the risk of pneumothorax:

(a) The use of positive end expiratory pressure
(b) Tachypnoea
(c) The presence of a bulla in the lung
(d) Addiction to narcotic analgesics

308. Rheumatic fever in early life can cause:

(a) Liver damage
(b) Brain damage
(c) Damage to peripheral nerves
(d) Damage to the heart valves

309. Haemophilia:

(a) Can cause severe pain from bleeding into joints
(b) Is genetically inherited
(c) Can be cured by drug treatment
(d) Is more common in the elderly

310. The cause of death in typhoid fever is usually:

(a) Severe septicaemia
(b) Disorders of the blood
(c) Severe fluid depletion
(d) Brain haemorrhages

311. The Glasgow Coma Scale utilizes the following signs:

(a) Eye opening
(b) Verbal response
(c) Best motor response
(d) Muscle tone

312. Oxygen can be given by mask to patients suffering from severe chronic bronchitis. The safest percentage of oxygen to give in the immediate care situation is:

(a) 21%
(b) 24%
(c) 36%
(d) 48%

313. Carbon monoxide poisoning usually produces:

(a) A greyish hue to the skin
(b) Central cyanosis
(c) Severe hypoxaemia
(d) Renal failure

314. Which of the following factors increases the risk of deep vein thrombosis:

(a) Bed rest
(b) Anaemia
(c) Obesity
(d) Physiotherapy

315. Which of the following drugs is best avoided in patients with penetrating eye injuries:

(a) Thiopentone
(b) Suxamethonium
(c) Etomidate
(d) Pancuronium

316. Signs of deep vein thrombosis in the leg include:

(a) Swelling in the affected leg
(b) Pain on pressing the calf muscles
(c) Wasting of the muscles in the leg
(d) Loss of arterial pulses in the affected leg

317. Features of overdosage of local anaesthetic agents include:

(a) Fits
(b) Increase in abdominal tone
(c) Hypotension
(d) Tinnitus (ringing in the ears)

318. Which of these anaesthetic agents has the fastest onset of action:

(a) Halothane
(b) Trichlorethylene
(c) Cyclopropane
(d) Enflurane

319. The Lack Circuit behaves physically like a:

(a) Magill Circuit
(b) Bain Circuit
(c) Water's Circuit
(d) T-Piece Circuit

320. A suitable endotracheal tube for an average child of 8 years would have an internal diameter of:

(a) 4 mm
(b) 5·5 mm
(c) 6·5 mm
(d) 8 mm

321. Which of the following is likely to lead to bleeding from the gastric mucosa:

(a) The presence of a nasogastric tube
(b) Repeated doses of systemic steroids
(c) Anticoagulant therapy
(d) Endotracheal intubation

322. The cement used in hip surgery (methylmethacrylate) may cause:

(a) Pyrexia
(b) Hypotension
(c) Cyanosis
(d) Hyperventilation

323. The following are good indications for endotracheal intubation:

(a) Head and neck surgery
(b) Patient with a full stomach
(c) Use of positive pressure ventilation
(d) Day case surgery

324. Awake intubation is indicated in:

(a) Neonates
(b) Adolescents
(c) The elderly
(d) Children with acute epiglottitis

325. Sellick's Manoeuvre (cricoid pressure) is designed to prevent:

(a) Vomiting
(b) Regurgitation of stomach contents
(c) Tachycardia
(d) Bradycardia

326. The Bain Circuit is classified as:

(a) Mapleson A
(b) Mapleson B
(c) Mapleson C
(d) Mapleson D

327. Signs of respiratory obstruction following extubation may be due to:

(a) Laryngeal oedema
(b) Laryngeal spasm
(c) Subglottic oedema
(d) Inhaled foreign body

328. Treatment of convulsions consequent upon the inadvertent intravenous injection of local anaesthetic might include:

(a) Thiopentone
(b) Intravenous adrenaline
(c) Oxygen by positive pressure ventilation
(d) Mannitol

329. Subarachnoid (spinal) block with local analgesic drugs may be followed by:

(a) Headache
(b) Retention of urine
(c) Meningitis
(d) Nephritis

330. The Mackintosh laryngoscope:

(a) Is only suitable for neonates
(b) Has a curved blade
(c) Is especially made for a left-handed operator
(d) Is designed so that its tip lies in front of the epiglottis in use

331. When a laser beam is used in laryngeal surgery:

(a) The endotracheal tube must be protected with aluminium foil
(b) There is no contra-indication to the use of flammable anaesthetic agents and apparatus
(c) Personnel must wear protective eyeglasses
(d) There is no radiation danger to the pregnant patient

332. Perforated peptic ulcer is suggested by which of the following:

(a) Abdominal pain
(b) Localized tenderness in the right iliac fossa
(c) Passing of bright red blood per rectum
(d) Impending cardiovascular collapse

333. Penetrating injury to the globe of the eye is suggested by:

(a) An irregular pupil
(b) Loss of the normal anterior curvature of the eye
(c) Double vision
(d) Loss of feeling in the affected eye

334. Hypoxic drive becomes the normal stimulus to respiration at altitudes above:

(a) 100 m
(b) 300 m
(c) 1000 m
(d) 3000 m

335. Following severe burns to the lower leg, the following procedures should be carried out:

(a) Removal of shoes and socks
(b) Assessment of the peripheral pulse distal to the injury
(c) Comparison of colour and temperature between the right and left feet
(d) Immersion of the limb in warm water if the pulse is not felt

336. Treatment of the 'crush syndrome' might include:

(a) Restoration of circulating volume
(b) Administration of potassium intravenously
(c) Monitoring of central venous pressure
(d) Use of diuretics

337. The following are potential complications of oxygen therapy:

(a) Pulmonary tissue damage
(b) Damage behind the lens of the eye in neonates
(c) Ventilatory depression
(d) Pulmonary oedema

338. Mechanical ventilation usually involves tidal volumes of:

(a) 4–5 ml/kg
(b) 10–12 ml/kg
(c) 20–30 ml/kg
(d) 60–80 ml/kg

339. In the 'rules of nines' used in the assessment of burns, for an adult:

(a) The arm represents 9%
(b) Each side of the arm represents 9%
(c) Both arms represent 9%
(d) The perineum represents 18%

340. Of the following, the most efficient method of artificial respiration is:

(a) Expired air method (mouth to mouth)
(b) Bag and mask (applied properly)
(c) Holger–Neilsen method
(d) Sylvester's method

341. Following ingestion of turpentine the patient should:

(a) Be given a gastric washout
(b) Be given sodium bicarbonate to drink
(c) Be considered for dialysis
(d) Be admitted to hospital for observation

342. In the electrocardiogram:

(a) The P-wave represents ventricular contraction
(b) The QRS complex represents the ventricular recovery phase
(c) The normal P-wave is absent in atrial fibrillation
(d) A normal QRS complex is still seen in ventricular fibrillation

343. In diabetes mellitus:

(a) The patient always requires insulin
(b) The disease is due to failure of the part of the pancreas which produces pancreatic juice
(c) Is classified into 'juvenile' and 'maturity onset' types
(d) Is classified into exocrine and endocrine types

344. In haemorrhagic shock (hypovolaemia):

(a) The pulse is strong and bounding
(b) The stroke volume (volume of each heart beat) progressively increases
(c) Results in the preservation of skin blood flow at the expense of the brain
(d) Results in the preservation of blood flow to the brain at the expense of the kidney

345. Tetanus:

(a) Is due to a bacterial toxin
(b) Symptoms can be reversed with penicillin
(c) When fatal, death is due to asphyxia and exhaustion
(d) Causes cardiac arrest due to a toxic effect on the vagus nerve

346. In management of childbirth by critical care personnel:

(a) The cord should always be cut to prevent air embolus
(b) A pulsating cord indicates separation of the placenta
(c) The baby *must* be intubated if it is blue
(d) The placenta may be discarded immediately, before examination by doctor or midwife

347. Chronic bronchitis:

(a) Is often associated with emphysema
(b) May predispose to pneumonia
(c) Is characterized by a productive cough (sputum) throughout most of the year
(d) May lead to cyanosis

348. Pneumonia:

(a) Is always fatal
(b) May affect only small segments of the lung
(c) Often gives rise to pleurisy (sharp pain on inspiration)
(d) Is always caused by bacteria

349. Acute appendicitis:

(a) Tends to occur in the elderly
(b) Gives rise to pain which eventually localizes to the right lower quadrant of the abdomen
(c) May lead to peritonitis
(d) Is due to a viral infection

350. The Glasgow Coma scale

(a) Requires specialist training in neurological assessment
(b) Is based on eye opening, verbal response and tendon reflexes
(c) Involves three sections including motor and verbal responses
(d) Is not useful in head injuries

351. The most common cause of myocardial infarction is:

(a) Coronary thrombosis
(b) Coronary spasm
(c) Tuberculosis
(d) Aortic aneurysm

352. Chest pain due to myocardial ischaemia ('cardiac pain') characteristically:

(a) Lies behind the sternum
(b) Is colicky in nature
(c) Is relieved by exercise
(d) Is brought on by exercise

353. A cerebrovascular accident (stroke):

(a) Is usually fatal
(b) Is a common cause of unconsciousness
(c) Is a complication of high blood pressure
(d) May result in a speech impediment

354. Bronchial asthma:

(a) Always begins in childhood
(b) Is often due to allergy (hypersensitivity) to the house dust mite
(c) May have a family history
(d) Is never a fatal disease

355. During oligaemic (blood loss) shock the blood vessels in the skin are usually:

(a) Dilated
(b) Constricted
(c) Not changed
(d) Ruptured

356. An aortic aneurysm may present with:

(a) Severe back pain
(b) Cardiovascular collapse
(c) Incontinence of urine
(d) Haematemesis (vomiting blood)

357. Tingling or 'pins and needles' sensation in the limb of an injured patient should always alert you to the possibility of:

(a) Vascular damage
(b) Muscle injury
(c) Severed tendons
(d) Nerve damage

358. A patient with severe congestive cardiac failure will have:

(a) Shortness of breath
(b) Swelling of ankles
(c) Inability to lie down
(d) Green sputum

359. The heart rate may be irregular due to:

(a) Atrial fibrillation
(b) Sinus arrhythmia
(c) Sinus bradycardia
(d) Ventricular extra systoles

360. Oedema can be caused by:

(a) Excessive calcium intake
(b) Excessive plasma protein concentration
(c) A deficiency of potassium
(d) A deficiency of plasma proteins

361. Many patients display shortness of breath. This is known as:

(a) Orthopnoea
(b) Eupnoea
(c) Dyspnoea
(d) Hyperpnoea

362. The following are features of insulin overdose:

(a) Rapid onset
(b) Acetone smell on breath
(c) Rapid response to intravenous sugar
(d) Sweating

363. The indicator used in soda lime is:

(a) Phenol red
(b) Phenolphthalein
(c) Waxolene blue
(d) Litmus

364. An antistatic rubber is black due to impregnation with:

(a) Dye
(b) Copper
(c) Carbon
(d) Bismuth

365. Which of the following are steroids:

(a) Methylprednisolone
(b) Methylmethacrylate
(c) Methylamphetamine
(d) Methylcellulose

366. The following are signs of hypovolaemic shock:

(a) Pallor
(b) High blood pressure
(c) Rapid pulse
(d) Warm skin

367. The following are features of fainting:

(a) Pallor
(b) Rapid recovery after laying flat
(c) Strong pulse
(d) Hypotension

368. The following are causes of hypovolaemic shock:

(a) Bleeding
(b) Dehydration
(c) Drowning
(d) Burns

369. The following are causes of delayed stomach emptying:

(a) Shock
(b) Narcotic analgesics
(c) Trauma
(d) Oesophagitis

370. Which of the following artificial airways offers the most effective means of ventilation:

(a) Oropharyngeal airway
(b) Endotracheal tube
(c) Oesophageal obturator airway
(d) Oesophageal gastric tube airway

371. A patient who has swallowed a quantity of aspirin should:

(a) Be made to vomit
(b) Undergo gastric lavage
(c) Be admitted to hospital for observation
(d) Be given Fuller's earth via a gastric tube

372. Organophosphorus insecticides may prove fatal because they:

(a) Cause muscle paralysis
(b) Cause epileptic fits
(c) Cause bronchospasm
(d) Cause gastrointestinal haemorrhage

373. Which of the following is not a synthetic local analgesic agent:

(a) Bupivacaine
(b) Prilocaine
(c) Lignocaine
(d) Cocaine

374. Atrial fibrillation:

(a) Is a fatal condition
(b) May lead to embolus formation
(c) Is treated with digitalis
(d) May be abolished by d.c. shock

375. In asystole, the treatment includes:

(a) Defibrillation with 400 J
(b) Oxygen, given by positive pressure ventilation
(c) Intravenous adrenaline
(d) Calcium chloride intravenously

376. Treatment of a partial thickness burn to more than 20% of the body surface area in an adult should include:

(a) Analgesia with opiates
(b) Immediate transfusion with 2 litres of whole blood
(c) Infusion of electrolyte solution
(d) Application of topical antibiotics

377. The following drugs may be used to treat acute pulmonary oedema due to left ventricular failure:

(a) Hartmann's solution
(b) 8·4% sodium bicarbonate
(c) Frusemide injection
(d) Digitalis glycosides

378. 'Berry' aneurysms are found in the:

(a) Thorax
(b) Abdomen
(c) Skull
(d) Pelvis

379. Which of the following drugs would be of use in the treatment of status epilepticus:

(a) Diazepam
(b) Doxapram
(c) Metaclopromide
(d) Thiopentone

380. Which of the following names are associated with endotracheal tube connectors:

(a) Nosworthy
(b) Magill
(c) Rowbotham
(d) Boyle

381. Hypothermia:

(a) Causes a fast irregular pulse rate
(b) Causes poor peripheral circulation
(c) Has an increased incidence in neonates
(d) In severe cases can cause ventricular fibrillation

382. Status epilepticus is life threatening because:

(a) Fits can cause fractures to the long bones
(b) Of excessive blood loss from biting the tongue
(c) Of impaired respiratory function
(d) Inability to retain voluntary sphincter control

383. The only effective drug in the treatment of malignant hyperpyrexia is:

(a) Thiopentone sodium
(b) Chlorpromazine
(c) Ice-cold saline
(d) Dantrolene sodium

384. In epidural anaesthesia which of the following are commonly seen in the affected limbs:

(a) Vasodilatation of the peripheries
(b) Vasoconstriction of the peripheries
(c) Loss of motor control
(d) Sweating in the affected limb

385. 'Maturity-onset' diabetics:

(a) Usually require insulin
(b) Are often treated by diet alone
(c) Do not require medical supervision
(d) Do not suffer the complications of the disease such as eye and circulatory problems

386. Pre-eclampsia (toxaemia of pregnancy):

(a) Is due to bacterial infection
(b) Is diagnosed by looking for oedema, protein in the urine and elevated blood pressure
(c) Is helped by rest and sedation
(d) May require delivery of the baby to prevent convulsions

387. Hypothermia:

(a) Is most common at the extremes of age
(b) May result in cardiac arrest
(c) Prolongs the period of time following cardiac arrest in which the effects of cerebral hypoxia are reversible
(d) May be induced artificially for cardiac surgery

388. Tetanus:

(a) Is due to a Gram-negative bacterium
(b) Is due to a toxoid
(c) Untreated results in death from exhaustion and hypoxia
(d) Is due to a viral toxin

389. Epilepsy:

(a) May begin in childhood
(b) May be due to previous head injury
(c) Gives a characteristic appearance on the electroencephalogram (EEG)
(d) May be treated with certain barbiturate drugs

390. Stroke (cerebrovascular accident, CVA) can:

(a) Be due to a haemorrhage within the brain
(b) Be due to a clot in a cerebral vessel
(c) Follow atrial fibrillation
(d) Cause problems with blood pressure and breathing

391. Internal bleeding:

(a) Always becomes apparent sooner or later as 'revealed' haemorrhage
(b) May lead to hypotension and 'shock' with no visible blood loss
(c) Is self-limiting and requires no treatment
(d) Requires thorough investigation of the cause

392. All cases of chest injury must have a:

(a) Chest X-ray
(b) Cervical spine X-ray
(c) Cervical collar applied at site of accident
(d) Chest drain inserted

393. The following are causes of vaginal bleeding:

(a) Abortion
(b) Eclampsia
(c) Placenta praevia
(d) Retained placenta

394. The following are features of a grand mal epileptic fit:

(a) Tonic and clonic phases
(b) Biting tongue
(c) Cyanosis
(d) Incontinence

395. The following are signs of profound hypothermia:

(a) Hyperactivity
(b) Bradycardia
(c) Hypotension
(d) Slow breathing

396. The following are causes of hyperventilation:

(a) Aspirin overdose
(b) Hysteria
(c) Diabetic ketoacidosis
(d) Barbiturate overdose

397. Features of the crush syndrome are:

(a) Haemoglobinuria
(b) Crushed larynx
(c) Renal failure
(d) Immediate recovery following treatment with steroids

398. A partial thickness burn of 10% of body area in an adult:

(a) Is usually fatal
(b) Is painless
(c) Would benefit from intravenous analgesia with an opiate
(d) May lead to septicaemia from infection

399. Ingestion of a corrosive poison such as bleach should be treated by:

(a) Induction of vomiting
(b) Dilution of the corrosive with water
(c) Gastric lavage with charcoal
(d) Intravenous sodium thiosulphate

400. Barbiturates:

(a) Are the most common group of drugs involved in self-poisoning
(b) Are the safest among hypnotic drugs
(c) Interact dangerously with alcohol
(d) May cause respiratory depression

401. In a patient who collapses shortly after delivery of a baby the following diagnosis must be considered:

(a) Amniotic fluid embolus
(b) Pulmonary embolus
(c) Septicaemia
(d) Post-partum haemorrhage

402. 'Croup' is:

(a) Due to an infection
(b) Due to a congenital abnormality of the lower respiratory tract
(c) Affects only children of white (Caucasian) parents
(d) Always a mild disease

403. The infant larynx is:

(a) Narrowest at the vocal cords
(b) Narrowest at the cricoid cartilage
(c) Protected by a relatively large epiglottis compared to an adult
(d) Protected by less efficient reflexes than in the adult

404. Diabetics of the juvenile (insulin dependent) type:

(a) Have too much circulating insulin
(b) Produce normal amounts of insulin but it is ineffective at cellular level
(c) If untreated pass into coma from low blood sugar
(d) Have the smell of acetone on their breath in untreated diabetic coma

405. Crush injuries to the pelvis may lead to:

(a) Haematuria (blood in the urine)
(b) Pneumaturia (gas in the urine)
(c) Peritonitis
(d) Renal failure

406. Hyperglycaemia means:

(a) A low blood sugar level
(b) A low plasma calcium level
(c) A high blood sugar level
(d) Sugar in the urine

407. Tachypnoea is the term used to describe:

(a) Resistance to a drug's effects
(b) A slow heart rate
(c) A rapid respiratory rate
(d) Slow deep breathing

408. Stridor is often associated with:

(a) Laryngospasm
(b) Spasm of the sphincter of Oddi
(c) Inhaled foreign body
(d) Damage to the facial nerve

409. There is a profuse spontaneous nosebleed. The bleeding will best be stopped by:

(a) Lying down, head turned away from the side of the bleeding nostril
(b) Sitting up, slightly forward and pinching bridge of nose firmly
(c) Applying a cold compress to upper back to provoke reflex constriction of vessels
(d) Packing the nostril firmly with any convenient gauze or wick

410. Intra-operative blood loss can be most accurately measured by:

(a) Swab weighing
(b) Estimation 'by eye'
(c) Colorimetry
(d) Postoperative haemoglobin estimation

411. Which of the following conditions can cause chest pain:

(a) Intermittent claudication
(b) Myocardial infarction
(c) Pulmonary embolus
(d) Pneumonia

412. Which of the following statements are true:

(a) Swab checking eliminates the possibility of swabs being left in the wound
(b) Checking the operative site is unnecessary if it is already marked
(c) Checking of blood for donation should be undertaken by two people
(d) If the surgeon insists that the operative site marked is incorrect, this should not be questioned

413. Headache following spinal analgesia is:

(a) Due to CSF leak
(b) Alleviated by sitting or standing
(c) Minimized by an epidural saline drip
(d) Worse when fine gauge needles are used

414. The Magill circuit is a:

(a) Mapleson A circuit
(b) Mapleson B circuit
(c) Mapleson C circuit
(d) Mapleson D circuit

415. Which of the following can cause hypothermia:

(a) Atropinization (belladonna poisoning)
(b) Hypothyroidism
(c) Unconsciousness
(d) Hyperthyroidism

416. The Heimlich manoeuvre is used to:

(a) Expel foreign bodies from the larynx
(b) Pass an endotracheal tube in a difficult intubation
(c) Give artificial respiration
(d) Stabilize a fractured long bone

417. In a traumatized patient, the following are signs of developing adult respiratory distress syndrome (shock lung):

(a) Decreasing inflation pressures required to ventilate the lung
(b) Decreasing lung compliance (elasticity)
(c) Leakage of red cells into the alveoli
(d) Vomiting of blood

418. Acute epiglotitis in children:

(a) Is known as 'croup'
(b) Is due to an inhaled foreign body
(c) May be due to a viral infection
(d) May cause obstruction of the airway by the epiglottis

419. Stab wounds to the thorax are likely to result in:

(a) Haemothorax
(b) Haemopericardium
(c) Pneumothorax
(d) Haemoptysis (spitting blood)

420. Bleeding from the ear may indicate:

(a) Fracture of the stapes
(b) Basal skull fracture
(c) Trauma to the external auditory canal
(d) Aneurysm of the aorta

421. Which of the following conditions contra-indicates giving aspirin:

(a) Coronary thrombosis
(b) Peptic ulceration
(c) Ulcerative colitis
(d) Meningitis

422. Swelling occurs in inflammation because:

(a) Local sodium levels are increased
(b) Permeability of capillaries is increased
(c) Extra cells are present in the area
(d) Lymphatic drainage is impaired

423. Which of the following may occur in a patient as a result of prolonged bedrest:

(a) Accumulation of potassium in the muscle
(b) Loss of calcium from the bones
(c) Sodium retention in the kidneys
(d) Increased iron storage in the liver

424. After lumbar puncture, which of the following should a nurse encourage a patient to do:

(a) Get up and about immediately
(b) Sit up, supported by four pillows
(c) Lie flat in bed for 6–12 hours
(d) Lie prone for 12 hours

425. In lower neurone disease the muscle tone is usually:

(a) Unaffected
(b) Spastic
(c) Subject to periods of tonic and clonic spasticity
(d) Flaccid

426. The temperature of a baby's bath in degrees Celsius should be:

(a) 20
(b) 38
(c) 45
(d) 60

427. Blood stained cerebrospinal fluid in an unconscious patient is usually indicative of a:

(a) Extradural haemorrhage
(b) Subdural haemorrhage
(c) Subarachnoid haemorrhage
(d) Intra-cerebral haemorrhage

428. Otorhinorrhoea (fluid leak from the ears and nose) observed in a patient with a suspected fractured skull is significant because:

(a) The vestibular apparatus may be damaged
(b) Meningitis is a potential hazard
(c) The intra-cranial pressure may fall
(d) It indicates extensive brain damage

429. Because of its central role in co-ordinating complex motor activity damage to which of the following structures will result in jerky, unco-ordinated movement:

(a) Cerebrum
(b) Cerebellum
(c) Medulla oblongata
(d) Limbic system

430. When the heart doubles or trebles the number of systolic beats per minute, the condition is known as:

(a) Heart block
(b) Mitral stenosis
(c) Tachycardia
(d) Sinus bradycardia

431. The sounds that one hears when listening to the normal heart with a stethoscope are made by which of the following:

(a) The closing of the valves in each heart cycle
(b) The blood entering and leaving the heart
(c) The impulses travelling from the SA node to the Purkinje fibres
(d) The ventricles contracting and relaxing

432. Following operation, it is usual for patients to:

(a) Pass more urine than normal
(b) Pass less urine than normal
(c) Have no change in urine volume
(d) Pass no urine at all for 24 hours

433. Phaeochromocytoma (tumour of the adrenal medulla) causes:

(a) Complete destruction of the gland
(b) Hyposecretion of catecholamines
(c) Hypotension
(d) Hypersecretion of catecholamines

434. Common signs and symptoms of Addison's disease include:

(a) Generalized weakness, increased skin pigmentation, hypotension and emotional disturbances
(b) Buffalo hump, weight gain and skin striae
(c) Hyperglycemia, increased frequency of infections and polyuria
(d) Grotesque appearance, increased oiliness of skin and hair, headaches and impotence

435. When the atria are relaxed and receiving blood, which one of the following statements is correct:

(a) The ventricles are relaxed and the atrio-ventricular valves are closed
(b) The ventricles are contracting and the semilunar valves are closed
(c) The ventricles are contracting and the atrio-ventricular valves are open
(d) The ventricles are contracting and the atrio-ventricular valves are closed

436. If the extracellular fluid becomes hypotonic, water shifts:

(a) From the extracellular fluid into the intracellular fluid to equalize the water concentration through osmosis
(b) From the intracellular fluid into the extracellular fluid to equalize the water concentration through osmosis
(c) From the extracellular fluid into the intracellular fluid to equalize the water concentration through diffusion
(d) From the extracellular fluid into the intracellular fluid to equalize the water concentration through facilitated diffusion

437. Which of the following vitamins may be given to facilitate blood clotting:

(a) Vitamin B complex
(b) Vitamin E
(c) Vitamin D
(d) Vitamin K

438. Dupuytren's contracture is:

(a) Remediable by surgery
(b) Caused by a virus
(c) A foot deformity
(d) A flexion deformity in the hand

439. In osteoporosis:

(a) There is an imbalance between bone formation and bone reabsorption
(b) Calcium is over-produced
(c) There is a progressive weakness of leg muscles
(d) Proteins are excreted in excessive amounts

440. In nursing a patient who has terminal cancer, the most important nursing goal is:

(a) Returning the patient to the community
(b) Preventing metastasis forming
(c) Encouraging the patient to expect to be cured
(d) Controlling the symptoms

441. A child is admitted to the paediatric ward clutching a small grubby blanket. Should you:

(a) Give the blanket to the mother to take home
(b) Let the child keep it by her
(c) Wash the blanket in disinfectant
(d) Put the blanket out of reach but not out of sight

442. Symptoms of myxoedema include:

(a) Profuse perspiration and slowing down of all activities
(b) Increased sensitivity to cold and thinning of the hair
(c) Fatigue and profuse perspiration
(d) Weight loss and inability to adapt to new situations

443. A patient with hyperthyroidism will complain of:

(a) Increased appetite with weight gain
(b) Decreased appetite with weight loss
(c) Increased appetite with weight gain
(d) Decreased appetite with weight gain

444. The proximal convoluted tubules:

(a) Reabsorb most of the water and salts of the glomerular filtrate
(b) Reabsorb most of the glucose of the glomerular filtrate
(c) Contain the cells which secrete renin
(d) Are the main target cells for ADH

445. BCG vaccine:

(a) Contains dead bacilli
(b) Is an effective antidote to tuberculosis
(c) Is given to persons who have a positive reaction to tuberculin
(d) Is given to persons who have a negative reaction to tuberculin

446. The following drug is used specifically in the treatment of Parkinson's disease:

(a) Laevodopa
(b) Methyldopa
(c) Lorazepam
(d) Primidone

447. After initial digitalization which of the following doses of digoxin is likely to be prescribed as a maintenance dose in a 70 kg adult of 50 years:

(a) 0·025 mg daily
(b) 0·25 mg daily
(c) 2·5 mg daily
(d) 25 mg daily

448. Postoperative nausea and vomiting may be treated with:

(a) Metoclopromide
(b) Cyclizine
(c) Doxapram
(d) Neostigmine

449. A patient suffering from leukaemia is often given a transfusion of packed cells to relieve anaemia. Packed cells are given rather than whole blood in order:

(a) To reduce the volume of serum given, thereby lessening the risk of hepatitis
(b) To minimize the infusion of donor antibodies
(c) To limit the transfusion time by reducing the volume of blood to be infused
(d) To effect cell replacement whilst avoiding unnecessary fluid replacement

450. Which of the following agglutinogens will be present in the serum of an individual with A (Rhesus positive) blood group:

(a) Anti-A
(b) Anti-B
(c) Anti-A and anti-B
(d) None

451. In many instances a patient suffering from rheumatic fever will give a history of a recent infection indicative of a probable relationship between the disease and:

(a) Coxsackie virus
(b) Haemolytic streptococci
(c) *Staphylococcus aureus*
(d) Non-haemolytic streptococci

452. Following a head injury due to a fall from a horse:

(a) The period of unconsciousness is of no great significance to the final outcome.
(b) The absence of a fracture on skull X-ray eliminates any serious consequences
(c) Bleeding from the nose is of no significance
(d) Bleeding from the ear is of no significance

453. Patients prior to sub-total thyroidectomy are usually prescribed a saturated solution of potassium iodide, the primary reason being that the drug helps to:

(a) Reduce the vascularity of the gland
(b) Decrease the progression of exophthalmos
(c) Decrease the body's ability to store thyroxine
(d) Increase the body's ability to store thyroxine

454. A patient's blood pressure on admission was 120/80 mmHg. Following surgery the pulse pressure increases. Which of the following readings illustrates a pulse pressure greater than the original:

(a) 100/60 mmHg
(b) 110/90 mmHg
(c) 140/100 mmHg
(d) 160/100 mmHg

455. A complication arising from inadequate mouth care in a patient with agranulocytosis is thrush, this condition is caused by:

(a) *Staphylococcus aureus*
(b) *Candida albicans*
(c) *Staphylococcus albus*
(d) *Clostridium welchii*

456. Which of the following is most likely to induce an angina pectoris attack:

(a) Eating a heavy meal
(b) Prolonged inactivity
(c) A warm environment
(d) Physical exercise

457. A baby had an Apgar score of 8 at 1 minute and 10 at 5 minutes. This Apgar score indicates that the infant's condition is:

(a) Poor
(b) Fair
(c) Good
(d) Critical

458. Coupling of the heart beat when a premature systole and compensatory pause follow each normal beat is called:

(a) Paroxysmal tachycardia
(b) Atrial flutter
(c) Extra systole
(d) Pulsus bigeminus

459. The pain of myocardial infarction differs from that of angina in that it is:

(a) Intermittent in nature
(b) More responsive to rest
(c) Rarely relieved by rest
(d) Less likely to radiate

460. The hormone which brings about changes in the female at puberty is:

(a) Progesterone
(b) Prolactin
(c) Oestrogen
(d) Oxytocin

461. Of the following complications, for which should the nurse be particularly alert when a patient has had spinal anaesthesia:

(a) Hypotension
(b) Convulsions
(c) Renal shutdown
(d) Urinary retention

462. Which of the following types of white blood cells is concerned with allergic response:

(a) Lymphocytes
(b) Neutrophils
(c) Monocytes
(d) Eosinophils

463. The acetylcholine released at the motor end-plates of skeletal muscle stimulates:

(a) Muscle relaxation
(b) Muscle paralysis
(c) Muscle contraction
(d) Muscle recoil

464. Lacteals function in the absorption of one of the following substances:

(a) Amino acids
(b) Carbohydrates
(c) Protein
(d) Fats

465. A benign tumour of fat is called a:

(a) Leiomyoma
(b) Liposarcoma
(c) Lipoma
(d) Mesothelioma

466. Patients with congestive cardiac failure are usually nursed sitting up and well supported by pillows. The purpose of this position is:

(a) To make breathing easier
(b) To increase the arterial blood pressure
(c) To encourage the movement of fluid from the lungs
(d) To increase the venous blood pressure

467. Paroxysmal attacks of hypertension are most likely to be due to which one of the following:

(a) Carcinoma of the kidney
(b) Phaeochromocytoma (tumour of adrenal medulla)
(c) Coronary artery disease
(d) Obstruction of the renal artery

468. The commonest causative organism of impetigo is:

(a) Staphylococcus
(b) Streptococcus
(c) Pseudomonas
(d) Clostridium

469. In a patient with chronic bronchitis the stimulus to breathe is:

(a) Rising level of CO_2 in the blood
(b) Shortage of O_2
(c) Falling potassium level
(d) The level of nitrogen in blood

470. An infant is admitted to the ward having had a convulsion. This is most likely to be due to:

(a) A subnormal body temperature
(b) Hysteria
(c) Apoplexy
(d) A raised body temperature

471. Which of the following urinary signs is most likely to occur when glomerular filtration is impaired as a result of shock:

(a) Reduced urinary output
(b) Increased urinary output
(c) Reduced pH level
(d) Increased pH level

472. A volvulus is the term given to the intestines when:

(a) It twists on itself causing an obstruction
(b) It folds in on itself forming a narrowing of the lumen
(c) It loses muscle tone and peristaltic action
(d) There is a sequence of enlargement and narrowing of the lumen

473. The immediate treatment for acute retention of urine is:

(a) Prostatectomy
(b) Catheterization
(c) Bladder washout
(d) Intravenous injection of diuretics

474. Which of the following is in the groin:

(a) Hiatus hernia
(b) Epigastric hernia
(c) Inguinal hernia
(d) Femoral hernia

475. Which of the following is a feature in prostatitis:

(a) Frequency of micturition
(b) Anuria
(c) Glycosuria
(d) Polyuria

476. Repair of an adult hernia is known as:

(a) Herniolysis
(b) Herniorrhapy
(c) Hernioplasty
(d) Herniectomy

477. Crohn's disease can be known as one of the following conditions:

(a) Regional ileitis
(b) Relapsing fever
(c) Remittent incontinence
(d) Paralytic ileus

478. A carcinogenic compound is one that:

(a) Is used to attempt to effect a cure for cancer
(b) Can detect the presence of cancer
(c) Delays the growth and spread of cancer
(d) Is thought to cause cancer

479. The normal amount of urine produced each day by a 70 kg man is one of the following:

(a) 200 ml
(b) 500 ml
(c) 1500 ml
(d) 5000 ml

480. After laparotomy recognized postoperative complications are:

(a) A paralytic ileus
(b) Facial oedema
(c) Haemorrhage from the wound
(d) Pancreatitis

481. The approximate amount of blood entering the kidneys each minute (cardiac output 5 litres/min) is:

(a) 800 ml
(b) 1800 ml
(c) 200 ml
(d) 1200 ml

482. The symptoms of nausea and vomiting in a patient suffering from chronic renal failure are due to the accumulation of:

(a) The end products of fat metabolism in the blood stream
(b) The end product of carbohydrate metabolism in the blood stream
(c) The end product of protein metabolism in the blood stream
(d) Ketone bodies in the blood stream

483. In coronary thrombosis there is usually a marked rise in:

(a) The level of urea in the blood
(b) The level of lymphocytes in the blood
(c) The level of transaminase in the blood
(d) The level of alkaline phosphatase in the blood

484. In the event of the development of aortic incompetence and in the absence of other valvular lesions, which chamber of the heart will enlarge (hypertrophy) first:

(a) Left atrium
(b) Left ventricle
(c) Right atrium
(d) Right ventricle

485. The correct term for a weak bulge in an artery wall is known as one of the following:

(a) An aneurysm
(b) An embolism
(c) A varicose vein
(d) An atheroma

486. The correct term for repair of a perforated eardrum is:

(a) Myringoplasty
(b) Myringotomy
(c) Turbinectomy
(d) Arthroplasty

487. Red bone marrow is found in:

(a) Cancellous tissue
(b) Compact tissue
(c) Haversian canals
(d) Periosteum

488. Which one of the following is *not* a mechanism by which the body loses heat:

(a) Insensible water loss
(b) Radiation
(c) Conduction
(d) Vaso-constriction via sympathetic NS

489. Difficulty in speaking coherently is known as:

(a) Dysphagia
(b) Dysphasia
(c) Dysplasia
(d) Dyspepsia

490. In which of the following sites in the adult are erythrocytes manufactured in the greatest numbers:

(a) Spleen
(b) Liver
(c) Reticulo-endothelial system
(d) Bone marrow

491. Hypoglycaemia is a blood sugar level which has fallen too low. One of the earliest features is:

(a) A feeling of dryness in the mouth
(b) Air hunger
(c) Extreme thirst
(d) Mental confusion

492. Which of the following is true of the kidneys:

(a) They are inside the peritoneum
(b) They are both at the same level
(c) The right kidney is lower than the left
(d) The lower pole of left kidney reaches the umbilicus

493. Which of the following statements is true of the right main bronchus in the adult:

(a) It is much larger (in diameter) than the left main bronchus
(b) It is longer than the left main bronchus
(c) It lies more vertically than the left bronchus
(d) It has more cilia than the left main bronchus

494. Substances from the blood enter the nephron due to one of the following processes:

(a) Osmosis
(b) Diffusion
(c) Direct contact between blood and the nephron
(d) Filtration under pressure from capillaries

495. Oxygen diffuses from the alveoli into the blood stream because:

(a) Oxygen pressure in the alveolar air is greater than in the venous blood
(b) Oxygen pressure in the alveolar air is less than in the venous blood
(c) The oxygen pressure in the tissues is high
(d) Oxygen pressure in the alveolar air is equal to that in the venous blood

496. A person suspected of sustaining concussion must be:

(a) Kept awake and walking about
(b) Given a mild sedative and allowed to sleep
(c) Kept under neurological observation
(d) Given narcotic analgesics

497. Which of the following signs is of no use in assessing a grossly shocked patient following severe blood loss:

(a) The blood pressure
(b) The pulse
(c) The degree of sweating
(d) The central venous pressure

498. Following injection treatment for varicose veins the patient should be instructed to wear a leg support:

(a) When standing for a prolonged period
(b) During the day
(c) When the legs ache
(d) Day and night

499. Which of the following diets will a patient suffering from thyrotoxicosis require:

(a) Fat free diet
(b) High calorie diet
(c) Low protein diet
(d) 1000 calorie diet

500. Abdominal pain and vomiting in a 10-year-old child:

(a) Might be the first symptom of diabetes
(b) May be a manifestation of the same allergic phenomenon causing asthma and migraine
(c) May be due to a throat infection
(d) Will always require the placement of a nasogastric tube

Answers

1. (a) True	(b) False	(c) False	(d) False
2. (a) False	(b) False	(c) True	(d) False
3. (a) False	(b) False	(c) True	(d) False
4. (a) False	(b) False	(c) True	(d) False
5. (a) False	(b) False	(c) True	(d) False
6. (a) True	(b) True	(c) True	(d) False
7. (a) True	(b) True	(c) False	(d) True
8. (a) True	(b) False	(c) False	(d) False
9. (a) False	(b) False	(c) True	(d) False
10. (a) False	(b) False	(c) False	(d) True
11. (a) False	(b) True	(c) False	(d) False
12. (a) False	(b) True	(c) False	(d) False
13. (a) True	(b) False	(c) False	(d) True
14. (a) False	(b) False	(c) True	(d) True
15. (a) True	(b) False	(c) True	(d) False
16. (a) False	(b) True	(c) False	(d) False
17. (a) False	(b) False	(c) False	(d) True
18. (a) False	(b) False	(c) False	(d) True
19. (a) True	(b) False	(c) True	(d) True
20. (a) False	(b) False	(c) True	(d) False
21. (a) True	(b) True	(c) False	(d) True
22. (a) True	(b) False	(c) True	(d) False
23. (a) True	(b) False	(c) True	(d) True
24. (a) False	(b) False	(c) False	(d) False

25. (a) True (b) False (c) False (d) False
26. (a) False (b) False (c) False (d) True
27. (a) True (b) True (c) True (d) False
28. (a) False (b) True (c) False (d) False
29. (a) False (b) False (c) True (d) False
30. (a) False (b) False (c) False (d) True
31. (a) False (b) True (c) False (d) False
32. (a) False (b) True (c) False (d) False
33. (a) False (b) True (c) False (d) False
34. (a) False (b) False (c) True (d) False
35. (a) False (b) False (c) True (d) False
36. (a) False (b) True (c) False (d) True
37. (a) True (b) True (c) True (d) False
38. (a) False (b) True (c) False (d) False
39. (a) True (b) False (c) True (d) True
40. (a) False (b) False (c) True (d) False
41. (a) False (b) True (c) False (d) False
42. (a) False (b) False (c) True (d) False
43. (a) False (b) True (c) False (d) False
44. (a) True (b) True (c) True (d) True
45. (a) True (b) False (c) False (d) False
46. (a) False (b) False (c) True (d) False
47. (a) True (b) True (c) True (d) False
48. (a) True (b) False (c) False (d) False
49. (a) True (b) False (c) False (d) False
50. (a) False (b) False (c) False (d) True
51. (a) False (b) False (c) False (d) True
52. (a) False (b) True (c) False (d) True
53. (a) False (b) False (c) True (d) False
54. (a) False (b) False (c) False (d) True
55. (a) True (b) False (c) False (d) True
56. (a) True (b) False (c) True (d) True
57. (a) True (b) True (c) True (d) False
58. (a) False (b) False (c) False (d) True
59. (a) True (b) False (c) False (d) False
60. (a) True (b) True (c) False (d) False
61. (a) False (b) False (c) False (d) True
62. (a) False (b) False (c) False (d) True

63. (a) False (b) False (c) False (d) True
64. (a) False (b) False (c) False (d) True
65. (a) True (b) True (c) False (d) True
66. (a) False (b) False (c) True (d) False
67. (a) False (b) True (c) True (d) False
68. (a) True (b) False (c) False (d) False
69. (a) True (b) True (c) True (d) False
70. (a) False (b) True (c) False (d) False
71. (a) False (b) True (c) False (d) False
72. (a) True (b) True (c) True (d) True
73. (a) False (b) False (c) True (d) False
74. (a) False (b) False (c) True (d) False
75. (a) False (b) True (c) False (d) True
76. (a) False (b) False (c) True (d) False
77. (a) False (b) False (c) False (d) True
78. (a) True (b) True (c) False (d) False
79. (a) True (b) False (c) False (d) False
80. (a) False (b) True (c) False (d) False
81. (a) False (b) True (c) False (d) True
82. (a) False (b) True (c) False (d) False
83. (a) False (b) True (c) True (d) False
84. (a) False (b) False (c) True (d) False
85. (a) True (b) False (c) True (d) False
86. (a) True (b) False (c) True (d) False
87. (a) True (b) False (c) False (d) False
88. (a) False (b) True (c) False (d) False
89. (a) True (b) True (c) True (d) True
90. (a) False (b) True (c) False (d) False
91. (a) False (b) True (c) False (d) True
92. (a) False (b) False (c) False (d) True
93. (a) True (b) True (c) False (d) False
94. (a) False (b) True (c) False (d) False
95. (a) True (b) True (c) True (d) True
96. (a) False (b) False (c) False (d) False
97. (a) False (b) True (c) False (d) True
98. (a) False (b) False (c) False (d) True
99. (a) True (b) True (c) True (d) False
100. (a) False (b) True (c) False (d) False

101. (a) True (b) False (c) False (d) False
102. (a) False (b) False (c) True (d) False
103. (a) True (b) False (c) True (d) True
104. (a) True (b) False (c) False (d) False
105. (a) False (b) False (c) False (d) True
106. (a) True (b) False (c) True (d) False
107. (a) True (b) False (c) False (d) False
108. (a) True (b) False (c) True (d) True
109. (a) False (b) False (c) True (d) False
110. (a) False (b) True (c) True (d) False
111. (a) False (b) False (c) False (d) True
112. (a) False (b) False (c) True (d) False
113. (a) True (b) True (c) True (d) True
114. (a) True (b) False (c) False (d) False
115. (a) False (b) False (c) True (d) False
116. (a) False (b) True (c) False (d) True
117. (a) True (b) False (c) False (d) False
118. (a) True (b) False (c) False (d) True
119. (a) False (b) True (c) False (d) False
120. (a) False (b) True (c) True (d) False
121. (a) False (b) True (c) False (d) False
122. (a) True (b) False (c) True (d) False
123. (a) True (b) False (c) False (d) True
124. (a) False (b) True (c) False (d) True
125. (a) True (b) True (c) True (d) True
126. (a) True (b) True (c) True (d) True
127. (a) False (b) False (c) False (d) True
128. (a) False (b) False (c) True (d) True
129. (a) True (b) False (c) True (d) True
130. (a) False (b) False (c) True (d) False
131. (a) True (b) False (c) True (d) False
132. (a) False (b) True (c) True (d) False
133. (a) True (b) True (c) True (d) False
134. (a) True (b) False (c) False (d) True
135. (a) True (b) True (c) True (d) False
136. (a) False (b) True (c) True (d) False
137. (a) False (b) True (c) True (d) True
138. (a) False (b) True (c) True (d) False

139. (a) True (b) True (c) True (d) False
140. (a) True (b) False (c) False (d) False
141. (a) False (b) True (c) False (d) False
142. (a) False (b) True (c) False (d) False
143. (a) False (b) True (c) False (d) True
144. (a) False (b) True (c) False (d) False
145. (a) False (b) False (c) True (d) False
146. (a) True (b) False (c) False (d) False
147. (a) False (b) False (c) True (d) False
148. (a) False (b) False (c) True (d) True
149. (a) False (b) True (c) False (d) False
150. (a) True (b) True (c) True (d) True
151. (a) False (b) False (c) False (d) True
152. (a) False (b) True (c) False (d) False
153. (a) True (b) True (c) True (d) True
154. (a) False (b) False (c) False (d) True
155. (a) False (b) True (c) True (d) True
156. (a) False (b) False (c) True (d) False
157. (a) True (b) False (c) False (d) True
158. (a) True (b) False (c) False (d) False
159. (a) False (b) True (c) True (d) True
160. (a) False (b) False (c) True (d) False
161. (a) False (b) False (c) False (d) True
162. (a) True (b) True (c) False (d) True
163. (a) False (b) False (c) True (d) False
164. (a) True (b) False (c) True (d) True
165. (a) True (b) True (c) False (d) True
166. (a) True (b) True (c) False (d) True
167. (a) True (b) False (c) True (d) True
168. (a) False (b) False (c) False (d) True
169. (a) True (b) True (c) False (d) True
170. (a) False (b) False (c) True (d) False
171. (a) True (b) False (c) False (d) True
172. (a) True (b) True (c) True (d) True
173. (a) True (b) False (c) True (d) True
174. (a) True (b) True (c) False (d) False
175. (a) True (b) True (c) False (d) True
176. (a) True (b) False (c) False (d) True

177.	(a) True	(b) True	(c) True	(d) False
178.	(a) False	(b) False	(c) True	(d) True
179.	(a) True	(b) False	(c) True	(d) True
180.	(a) True	(b) False	(c) True	(d) True
181.	(a) True	(b) True	(c) True	(d) False
182.	(a) True	(b) True	(c) False	(d) False
183.	(a) False	(b) False	(c) True	(d) True
184.	(a) False	(b) True	(c) False	(d) False
185.	(a) True	(b) False	(c) True	(d) False
186.	(a) True	(b) False	(c) True	(d) True
187.	(a) False	(b) False	(c) False	(d) True
188.	(a) False	(b) False	(c) True	(d) False
189.	(a) True	(b) True	(c) False	(d) True
190.	(a) False	(b) True	(c) False	(d) False
191.	(a) False	(b) False	(c) False	(d) True
192.	(a) False	(b) False	(c) False	(d) False
193.	(a) False	(b) False	(c) True	(d) True
194.	(a) True	(b) False	(c) True	(d) False
195.	(a) True	(b) True	(c) True	(d) False
196.	(a) False	(b) True	(c) False	(d) True
197.	(a) False	(b) True	(c) False	(d) True
198.	(a) False	(b) False	(c) False	(d) True
199.	(a) True	(b) True	(c) False	(d) True
200.	(a) True	(b) False	(c) False	(d) True
201.	(a) True	(b) True	(c) False	(d) True
202.	(a) True	(b) True	(c) True	(d) False
203.	(a) True	(b) True	(c) True	(d) False
204.	(a) False	(b) True	(c) False	(d) False
205.	(a) True	(b) True	(c) False	(d) True
206.	(a) True	(b) False	(c) True	(d) False
207.	(a) True	(b) True	(c) False	(d) False
208.	(a) True	(b) True	(c) False	(d) False
209.	(a) True	(b) False	(c) False	(d) False
210.	(a) False	(b) True	(c) True	(d) False
211.	(a) False	(b) True	(c) True	(d) False
212.	(a) True	(b) False	(c) True	(d) True
213.	(a) False	(b) False	(c) True	(d) False
214.	(a) True	(b) False	(c) False	(d) True

215. (a) True (b) True (c) True (d) True
216. (a) False (b) False (c) True (d) False
217. (a) True (b) False (c) False (d) True
218. (a) False (b) False (c) True (d) True
219. (a) False (b) False (c) True (d) True
220. (a) False (b) False (c) False (d) False
221. (a) False (b) True (c) True (d) False
222. (a) True (b) True (c) True (d) True
223. (a) True (b) True (c) False (d) True
224. (a) False (b) True (c) True (d) False
225. (a) True (b) False (c) False (d) False
226. (a) False (b) True (c) True (d) False
227. (a) True (b) True (c) True (d) False
228. (a) False (b) True (c) False (d) False
229. (a) True (b) True (c) True (d) True
230. (a) True (b) False (c) False (d) True
231. (a) True (b) False (c) True (d) True
232. (a) True (b) True (c) True (d) True
233. (a) True (b) True (c) True (d) True
234. (a) True (b) True (c) True (d) True
235. (a) True (b) True (c) True (d) True
236. (a) True (b) True (c) False (d) True
237. (a) True (b) True (c) True (d) False
238. (a) True (b) False (c) False (d) True
239. (a) False (b) False (c) True (d) False
240. (a) True (b) False (c) False (d) False
241. (a) False (b) False (c) False (d) True
242. (a) False (b) False (c) True (d) False
243. (a) True (b) True (c) True (d) False
244. (a) False (b) False (c) False (d) True
245. (a) False (b) False (c) True (d) True
246. (a) False (b) True (c) True (d) False
247. (a) True (b) False (c) False (d) True
248. (a) False (b) False (c) False (d) True
249. (a) False (b) False (c) True (d) False
250. (a) False (b) True (c) False (d) False
251. (a) True (b) True (c) True (d) True
252. (a) False (b) False (c) False (d) True

253.	(a) False	(b) True	(c) False	(d) False
254.	(a) False	(b) False	(c) False	(d) True
255.	(a) False	(b) True	(c) False	(d) False
256.	(a) False	(b) True	(c) False	(d) False
257.	(a) True	(b) True	(c) False	(d) False
258.	(a) True	(b) True	(c) True	(d) False
259.	(a) True	(b) True	(c) True	(d) False
260.	(a) True	(b) False	(c) False	(d) True
261.	(a) False	(b) False	(c) True	(d) False
262.	(a) True	(b) True	(c) False	(d) True
263.	(a) True	(b) True	(c) True	(d) False
264.	(a) True	(b) False	(c) True	(d) False
265.	(a) False	(b) True	(c) False	(d) False
266.	(a) False	(b) True	(c) False	(d) False
267.	(a) False	(b) False	(c) True	(d) False
268.	(a) True	(b) False	(c) True	(d) False
269.	(a) False	(b) False	(c) True	(d) False
270.	(a) True	(b) False	(c) True	(d) True
271.	(a) False	(b) True	(c) False	(d) False
272.	(a) True	(b) True	(c) True	(d) True
273.	(a) True	(b) False	(c) False	(d) False
274.	(a) True	(b) True	(c) False	(d) False
275.	(a) True	(b) True	(c) False	(d) False
276.	(a) True	(b) True	(c) False	(d) False
277.	(a) True	(b) True	(c) True	(d) True
278.	(a) True	(b) True	(c) True	(d) False
279.	(a) True	(b) True	(c) True	(d) False
280.	(a) True	(b) True	(c) False	(d) False
281.	(a) True	(b) True	(c) True	(d) True
282.	(a) True	(b) True	(c) False	(d) False
283.	(a) True	(b) False	(c) False	(d) False
284.	(a) False	(b) False	(c) False	(d) True
285.	(a) True	(b) True	(c) True	(d) False
286.	(a) False	(b) True	(c) True	(d) True
287.	(a) True	(b) False	(c) True	(d) False
288.	(a) True	(b) True	(c) True	(d) True
289.	(a) False	(b) True	(c) True	(d) False
290.	(a) True	(b) True	(c) False	(d) True

291.	(a) False	(b) False	(c) True	(d) False
292.	(a) True	(b) False	(c) False	(d) False
293.	(a) False	(b) True	(c) False	(d) True
294.	(a) True	(b) False	(c) True	(d) True
295.	(a) False	(b) False	(c) False	(d) False
296.	(a) True	(b) False	(c) False	(d) False
297.	(a) False	(b) True	(c) False	(d) True
298.	(a) True	(b) True	(c) True	(d) True
299.	(a) True	(b) True	(c) True	(d) False
300.	(a) False	(b) False	(c) True	(d) True
301.	(a) True	(b) True	(c) False	(d) False
302.	(a) True	(b) False	(c) True	(d) False
303.	(a) True	(b) True	(c) True	(d) False
304.	(a) False	(b) True	(c) False	(d) False
305.	(a) True	(b) True	(c) True	(d) False
306.	(a) True	(b) True	(c) True	(d) False
307.	(a) True	(b) False	(c) True	(d) False
308.	(a) False	(b) False	(c) False	(d) True
309.	(a) True	(b) True	(c) False	(d) False
310.	(a) False	(b) False	(c) True	(d) False
311.	(a) True	(b) True	(c) True	(d) False
312.	(a) False	(b) True	(c) False	(d) False
313.	(a) False	(b) False	(c) True	(d) False
314.	(a) True	(b) False	(c) True	(d) False
315.	(a) False	(b) True	(c) False	(d) False
316.	(a) True	(b) True	(c) False	(d) False
317.	(a) True	(b) False	(c) True	(d) True
318.	(a) False	(b) False	(c) True	(d) False
319.	(a) True	(b) False	(c) False	(d) False
320.	(a) False	(b) False	(c) True	(d) False
321.	(a) True	(b) True	(c) True	(d) False
322.	(a) False	(b) True	(c) False	(d) False
323.	(a) True	(b) True	(c) True	(d) False
324.	(a) True	(b) False	(c) False	(d) False
325.	(a) False	(b) True	(c) False	(d) False
326.	(a) False	(b) False	(c) False	(d) True
327.	(a) True	(b) True	(c) True	(d) True
328.	(a) True	(b) False	(c) True	(d) False

329.	(a) True	(b) True	(c) True	(d) False
330.	(a) False	(b) True	(c) False	(d) True
331.	(a) True	(b) False	(c) True	(d) True
332.	(a) True	(b) False	(c) False	(d) True
333.	(a) True	(b) True	(c) False	(d) False
334.	(a) False	(b) False	(c) False	(d) True
335.	(a) True	(b) True	(c) True	(d) False
336.	(a) True	(b) False	(c) True	(d) True
337.	(a) True	(b) True	(c) True	(d) False
338.	(a) False	(b) True	(c) False	(d) False
339.	(a) True	(b) False	(c) False	(d) False
340.	(a) False	(b) True	(c) False	(d) False
341.	(a) False	(b) False	(c) False	(d) True
342.	(a) False	(b) False	(c) True	(d) False
343.	(a) False	(b) False	(c) True	(d) False
344.	(a) False	(b) False	(c) False	(d) True
345.	(a) True	(b) False	(c) True	(d) False
346.	(a) False	(b) False	(c) False	(d) False
347.	(a) True	(b) True	(c) True	(d) True
348.	(a) False	(b) True	(c) True	(d) False
349.	(a) False	(b) True	(c) True	(d) False
350.	(a) False	(b) False	(c) True	(d) False
351.	(a) True	(b) False	(c) False	(d) False
352.	(a) True	(b) False	(c) False	(d) True
353.	(a) False	(b) True	(c) True	(d) True
354.	(a) False	(b) True	(c) True	(d) False
355.	(a) False	(b) True	(c) False	(d) False
356.	(a) True	(b) True	(c) False	(d) False
357.	(a) True	(b) False	(c) False	(d) True
358.	(a) True	(b) True	(c) True	(d) False
359.	(a) True	(b) True	(c) False	(d) True
360.	(a) False	(b) False	(c) False	(d) True
361.	(a) False	(b) False	(c) True	(d) False
362.	(a) True	(b) False	(c) True	(d) True
363.	(a) False	(b) True	(c) False	(d) False
364.	(a) False	(b) False	(c) True	(d) False
365.	(a) True	(b) False	(c) False	(d) False
366.	(a) True	(b) False	(c) True	(d) False

367. (a) True (b) True (c) False (d) True
368. (a) True (b) True (c) False (d) True
369. (a) True (b) True (c) True (d) False
370. (a) False (b) True (c) False (d) False
371. (a) True (b) True (c) True (d) False
372. (a) True (b) False (c) False (d) False
373. (a) False (b) False (c) False (d) True
374. (a) False (b) True (c) True (d) True
375. (a) False (b) True (c) True (d) True
376. (a) True (b) False (c) True (d) False
377. (a) False (b) False (c) True (d) True
378. (a) False (b) False (c) True (d) False
379. (a) True (b) False (c) False (d) True
380. (a) True (b) True (c) True (d) False
381. (a) False (b) True (c) True (d) True
382. (a) False (b) False (c) True (d) False
383. (a) False (b) False (c) False (d) True
384. (a) True (b) False (c) True (d) False
385. (a) False (b) True (c) False (d) False
386. (a) False (b) True (c) True (d) True
387. (a) True (b) True (c) True (d) True
388. (a) False (b) False (c) True (d) False
389. (a) True (b) True (c) True (d) True
390. (a) True (b) True (c) True (d) True
391. (a) False (b) True (c) False (d) True
392. (a) True (b) True (c) True (d) False
393. (a) True (b) False (c) True (d) True
394. (a) True (b) True (c) True (d) True
395. (a) False (b) True (c) True (d) True
396. (a) True (b) True (c) True (d) False
397. (a) True (b) False (c) True (d) False
398. (a) False (b) False (c) True (d) True
399. (a) False (b) True (c) False (d) False
400. (a) False (b) False (c) True (d) True
401. (a) True (b) True (c) True (d) True
402. (a) True (b) False (c) False (d) False
403. (a) False (b) True (c) True (d) False
404. (a) False (b) False (c) False (d) True

405. (a) True (b) True (c) True (d) True
406. (a) False (b) False (c) True (d) False
407. (a) False (b) False (c) True (d) False
408. (a) True (b) False (c) True (d) False
409. (a) False (b) True (c) False (d) False
410. (a) False (b) False (c) True (d) False
411. (a) False (b) True (c) True (d) True
412. (a) False (b) False (c) True (d) False
413. (a) True (b) False (c) True (d) False
414. (a) True (b) False (c) False (d) False
415. (a) False (b) True (c) True (d) False
416. (a) True (b) False (c) False (d) False
417. (a) False (b) True (c) True (d) False
418. (a) False (b) False (c) True (d) True
419. (a) True (b) True (c) True (d) True
420. (a) False (b) True (c) True (d) False
421. (a) False (b) True (c) False (d) False
422. (a) False (b) True (c) False (d) False
423. (a) False (b) True (c) False (d) False
424. (a) False (b) False (c) True (d) False
425. (a) False (b) False (c) False (d) True
426. (a) False (b) True (c) False (d) False
427. (a) False (b) False (c) True (d) False
428. (a) False (b) True (c) False (d) False
429. (a) False (b) True (c) False (d) False
430. (a) False (b) False (c) True (d) False
431. (a) True (b) False (c) False (d) False
432. (a) False (b) True (c) False (d) False
433. (a) True (b) False (c) False (d) True
434. (a) True (b) False (c) False (d) False
435. (a) False (b) False (c) False (d) True
436. (a) True (b) False (c) False (d) False
437. (a) False (b) False (c) False (d) True
438. (a) True (b) False (c) False (d) True
439. (a) True (b) False (c) False (d) False
440. (a) False (b) False (c) False (d) True
441. (a) False (b) True (c) False (d) False
442. (a) False (b) True (c) False (d) False

443.	(a) False	(b) False	(c) True	(d) False
444.	(a) True	(b) False	(c) False	(d) False
445.	(a) False	(b) False	(c) False	(d) True
446.	(a) True	(b) False	(c) False	(d) False
447.	(a) False	(b) True	(c) False	(d) False
448.	(a) True	(b) True	(c) False	(d) False
449.	(a) False	(b) False	(c) False	(d) True
450.	(a) False	(b) True	(c) False	(d) False
451.	(a) False	(b) True	(c) False	(d) False
452.	(a) False	(b) False	(c) False	(d) False
453.	(a) True	(b) False	(c) False	(d) False
454.	(a) False	(b) False	(c) False	(d) True
455.	(a) False	(b) True	(c) False	(d) False
456.	(a) False	(b) False	(c) False	(d) True
457.	(a) False	(b) False	(c) True	(d) False
458.	(a) False	(b) False	(c) False	(d) True
459.	(a) False	(b) False	(c) True	(d) False
460.	(a) False	(b) False	(c) True	(d) False
461.	(a) True	(b) False	(c) False	(d) True
462.	(a) False	(b) False	(c) False	(d) True
463.	(a) False	(b) False	(c) True	(d) False
464.	(a) False	(b) False	(c) False	(d) True
465.	(a) False	(b) False	(c) True	(d) False
466.	(a) True	(b) False	(c) True	(d) False
467.	(a) False	(b) True	(c) False	(d) False
468.	(a) True	(b) False	(c) False	(d) False
469.	(a) False	(b) True	(c) False	(d) False
470.	(a) False	(b) False	(c) False	(d) True
471.	(a) True	(b) False	(c) False	(d) False
472.	(a) True	(b) False	(c) False	(d) False
473.	(a) False	(b) True	(c) False	(d) False
474.	(a) False	(b) False	(c) True	(d) True
475.	(a) True	(b) False	(c) False	(d) False
476.	(a) False	(b) True	(c) False	(d) False
477.	(a) True	(b) False	(c) False	(d) False
478.	(a) False	(b) False	(c) False	(d) True
479.	(a) False	(b) False	(c) True	(d) False
480.	(a) True	(b) False	(c) True	(d) False

481. (a) False (b) False (c) False (d) True
482. (a) False (b) False (c) True (d) False
483. (a) False (b) False (c) True (d) False
484. (a) False (b) True (c) False (d) False
485. (a) True (b) False (c) False (d) False
486. (a) True (b) False (c) False (d) False
487. (a) True (b) False (c) False (d) False
488. (a) False (b) False (c) False (d) True
489. (a) False (b) True (c) False (d) False
490. (a) False (b) False (c) False (d) True
491. (a) False (b) False (c) False (d) True
492. (a) False (b) False (c) True (d) False
493. (a) False (b) False (c) True (d) False
494. (a) False (b) False (c) False (d) True
495. (a) True (b) False (c) False (d) False
496. (a) False (b) False (c) True (d) False
497. (a) False (b) False (c) True (d) False
498. (a) False (b) False (c) False (d) True
499. (a) False (b) True (c) False (d) False
500. (a) True (b) True (c) True (d) False